Cannabis Compounds for Medical Conditions: An Evidence-Based Guide

James G. Williams, Ph.D.

Published by Page Notes, 2022.

While every precaution has been taken in the preparation of this book, the publisher assumes no responsibility for errors or omissions, or for damages resulting from the use of the information contained herein.

CANNABIS COMPOUNDS FOR MEDICAL CONDITIONS: AN EVIDENCE-BASED GUIDE

First edition. May 18, 2022.

ISBN: 979-8201020217

Written by James G. Williams, Ph.D..

Table of Contents

Acknowledgments

Thank you, Lauri Vrenda of the Thames Valley Dispensary, for introducing me to medical marijuana. Thank you, Marisa Wright, for your contribution to the cover design. Thank you, members of the Critique Circle, for feedback on the manuscript. Thank you, my son, Jameson, for your business advice and help with JavaScript. Thank you, Susan, for your love, patience, and support as my wife.

1: Introduction

Cannabis research papers are now coming out at the rate of about four thousand articles a year. The number is still larger if one includes articles on individual cannabis compounds. Most of these articles are medically relevant—many present convincing results in animal models of serious illnesses. There is a pressing need to get this vital research into the hands of patients, families, and physicians.

This book aims to present research about the medical benefits of cannabis compounds for physical and mental afflictions such as arthritis, intractable pain, Alzheimer's disease, schizophrenia, alcoholism, heart disease, and cancer. The word "research" is essential here. There have been many anecdotal stories of miraculous cannabis cures and treatments. In the web supplement to this book, medical claims are backed up by copious references to online medical research.

Topics covered in this introductory chapter include

1. A sketch of the book's main topics.
2. Types of cannabis compounds.
3. Types of medical evidence.
4. Procurement and use of cannabis compounds.
5. Comparison with previous work.
6. An introduction to the online supplement to this book.

1.1 Topics Covered

Chapter 2 explains the relationship between common forms of arthritis and inflammation. It then identifies cannabis compounds that can slow the progress of arthritis by reducing inflammation.

Chapter 3 covers pain and nausea: ordinary physical pain, including arthritis pain, neurological pain, and cancer pain.

Chapter 4 shows how cannabis compounds can help with Alzheimer's disease, epilepsy, traumatic brain injury, and other neurological conditions.

Chapter 5 discusses psychiatric conditions such as schizophrenia, depression, and post-traumatic stress disorder.

Chapter 6 is about compounds that can lead to addiction, including tobacco, alcohol, opioids, cocaine, and marijuana.

Chapter 7 presents what is known about how cannabis compounds affect strokes and cardiovascular conditions.

Chapter 8 discusses 17 types of cancer and presents the main cancer-fighting tasks performed by cannabis compounds.

Chapter 9 brings together all that is accomplished in Chapters 2 through 8. It gives a concise picture showing the relationship between cannabis compounds and the medical conditions studied. This information provides what strain developers need to develop new medically beneficial cannabis strains.

Appendix A lists the various cannabis compounds involved in treating medical conditions.

Appendix B discusses the ability of cannabis compounds to lower levels of inflammatory cytokines. Several chapters rely on Appendix B.

Appendix C is a short essay on the history of cannabis. It is included partly to show how cannabis terminology has evolved.

Appendix D is just a list of toxic compounds. This appendix is included as background for the discussion of neurological conditions.

Appendix E is a glossary of medical terms used in the book.

1.2 Types of Cannabis Compounds

Cannabis compounds fall into three main groups: cannabinoids, terpenes, and flavonoids. The quintessential cannabinoid, THC, achieves its effects primarily by interacting with the two cannabinoid receptors, CB1 and CB2. Cannabinoids are compounds that interact with the cannabinoid receptors or are structurally similar to compounds that do. The naturally occurring cannabinoids are found in the buds of female cannabis plants. The nine cannabinoids studied in this book are CBD, CBDA, THC, THCA, CBC, CBG, CBGA, THCV, and Δ8-THC.

Terpenes are light-weight oily compounds found not only in cannabis but in most other plants. Terpenes are construed to include oxidized terpenes called terpenoids. The following 21 terpenes are studied in this book:

borneol

camphene

d-limonene

eucalyptol

geraniol

guaiol

linalool

menthol

nerolidol

terpineol

terpinolene

valencene

α-bisabolol

α-humulene

α-pinene

α-terpinene

β-caryophyllene

β-caryophyllene oxide

β-eudesmol

β-pinene

γ-terpinene

Except for β-Caryophyllene, terpenes do not interact with the cannabinoid receptors.

In addition to cannabinoids and terpenes, cannabis plants also contain other compounds used in traditional folk medicine. They are found in cannabis roots, seeds, and sprouts. The flavonoid apigenin is an example. Cannabis testing laboratories do not yet test for flavonoids. They are beyond the scope of this book.

1.3 Types of Evidence

The following list presents seven types of evidence used in this book. Understanding evidence types is essential in studying cannabis compounds because there is precious little evidence resulting from large-scale double-blind, placebo-controlled studies of the sort used in the FDA's drug-approval process. This book aims to present available evidence accurately.

A *personal story* describes an illness, actions taken as part of treatment, and the outcome of the illness. Collecting someone's personal story may involve asking the following questions: How were you diagnosed? What medications have you taken? What cannabis strains or compounds were involved? How long before you saw results? Are you now symptom-free? If so, for how long? What factors may have contributed to the onset of your illness (e.g., age, gender, family history, herbicide exposure)? Do you have corroboration? These criteria come directly from studying patient stories.

A *Case Study* augments an individual's story with information about previous cases and explains why this case is significant. The case study recounts why the patient sought medical help and the basis for diagnosis (e.g., medical exam, blood tests, CT scans). It describes the duration and frequency of treatments, what the treatments were, how improvement was measured, and why treatments ended or are continuing. This description draws on the National Cancer Institute's *Compiling an NCI Best Case Submission*.

An *in vitro* study involves laboratory experiments with cells or tissues taken from plants, animals, or humans. A credible in vitro study begins with an exploration of scientific or medical background. It identifies specific objectives and hypotheses, describes materials and methods, and presents results. This description draws on Faggion's *Guidelines for Reporting Pre-Clinical In Vitro Studies on Dental Materials*.

Animal studies involve experiments on animals but may also include in vitro experiments. They predict which treatments are likely to work on humans and the likelihood of adverse effects. Animal studies involve ethical questions; see Lieu's *The Ethics of Animal Experimentation*.

Animal studies may involve *xenografts* which allow the study of human tissues hosted by animals. In many xenograft studies, it is possible to show that an experimental result is strictly the result of the human xenograft and is not influenced by the host animal.

Small-scale trials or *studies* divide patients into different treatment groups based on varying criteria. Depending on the design, researchers may need to know to which group a patient belongs. Such a study may be purely observational, as in the case of observed patient behaviors.

Large-scale studies involve a thousand subjects. They involve careful attention to experimental design to avoid experimental errors. Both small-scale and large-scale trials need to answer several questions: Did the study have a predetermined endpoint? How many study-related deaths and discontinuations were there? How did treatment affect the quality of life for those who completed the study? How many subjects were disease-free or had improved quality of life for a specified period following the study? See cancer.gov's *Levels of Evidence for Human Studies*.

Derivative documents include consensus statements, meta-analyses, expositions, and literature surveys. These are written to inform, raise awareness, or suggest new products and research. The validity of the presented evidence may be difficult to discern. For example, marijuana proponents and skeptics may rely on different inclusion criteria when performing meta-analyses.

In the absence of large-scale studies, the research results reported in this book are technically just hypotheses. What is true of one person's personal story *may* be true for another person. What is true of nude mice *may* be true for humans. And so forth.

In addition, there is the issue of replication. In medical science, the exact replication of an experiment is usually not attempted. Instead, related studies *may* get compatible results. Or not. In this book, when two studies conflict, both are reported.

Finally, there is the question of the reliability of individual results. Virtually all of the scientific results are from refereed research papers. A few of the published papers are from many years ago. They document the fact that some of the more significant facts have been known to the scientific community for quite some time.

1.4 Procurement and Use of Cannabis Compounds

The following chapters reveal, for selected medical conditions, cannabis compounds that may help. Having determined what cannabis compounds are relevant to a given medical condition, there are two ways to proceed: to obtain cannabis strains that feature the desired compounds or to buy the individual compounds directly.

Part 3 of Backes's *Cannabis Pharmacy* lists 50 strains of cannabis and gives an indication of what cannabis compounds are emphasized in each strain. Commercially available strains have been through many generations of strain development. None are the native indica or sativa strains found in the wild. However, choosing strains whose ancestry is mostly sativa or mostly indicia does afford some control over terpene content, as is shown in the following chart.

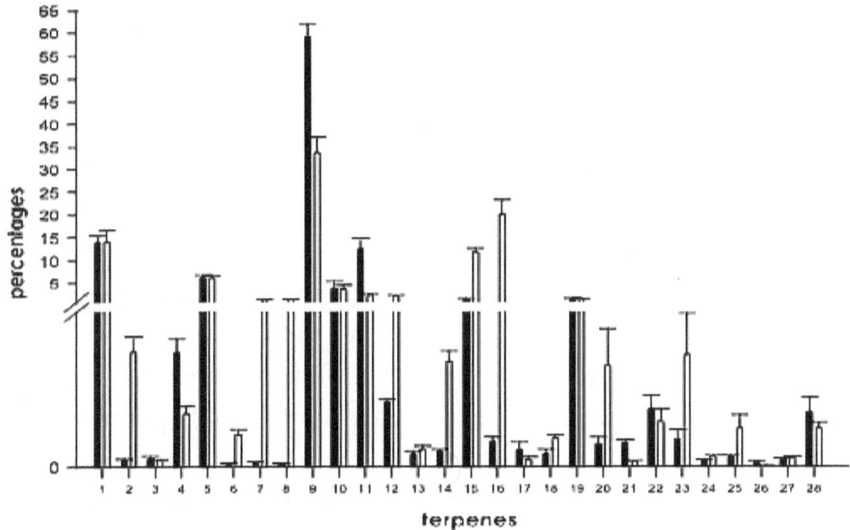

Legend. Mostly Indica=black bars, mostly Sativa=white bars. Break on Y-axis is 0.7. Numbers on X-axis refer to individual compounds: 1=α-pinene, 2=unk1, 3=unk2, 4=camphene, 5=β-pinene, 6=sabinene, 7=Δ-3-carene, 8=α-phellandrene, 9=β-myrcene, 10=α-terpinene, 11=limonene, 12=1.8 cineole, 13=γ-terpinene, 14=cis-β-ocimene, 15=trans-β-ocimene, 16=α-terpinolene, 17=unk3, 18=unk4, 19=β-caryophyllene, 20=unk5, 21=unk6, 22=unk7, 23=unk8, 24=unk9, 25=unk10, 26=unk11, 27=unk12, 28=unk13.

The above chart suggests that myrcene is the most abundant cannabis terpene. It has sedative properties and is responsible for the sedative effect of Indica cannabis strains. However, it is omitted from this book because the FDA has banned its use as a food additive on the grounds that it is carcinogenic.

Reputable online merchants provide independent third-party lab reports identifying the cannabis compounds contained in their products. States with medical cannabis programs commonly post third-party analyses of approved cannabis products. The state of

Connecticut, for example, posts these in an extensive online cannabis registry.

It is currently impossible to obtain a cannabis strain whose compounds are designed to handle a specific medical condition. However, work towards this goal has begun.

Aside from choosing a cannabis strain, the second option is selecting and consuming individual cannabis compounds. In addition to CBD, THC, CBDA, and THCA, several other cannabinoids are available over the internet. Pure cannabinoids are solids that are usually sold as tinctures dissolved in oil or alcohol. But water-soluble powders have been developed. A cannabinoid solution is more bioavailable and digests faster than a tincture. Several techniques for creating powders are in use, but the most common method is to create a powder whose particles are so fine that they stay in suspension when dissolved in water.

Individual terpenes are also available. They, too, are fat-soluble, but they are volatile oils rather than solids. They are also much more potent than cannabinoids. Some are used as seasonings, but most are not suited to ingestion. From Lawless's *The Encyclopedia of Essential Oils*, it is apparent that terpenes can be applied in any of the following ways:

dissolved in oils and lotions and applied to the skin

dissolved in massage oils and creams

infused into hot and cold compresses

released in vapor via evaporation

released in steam

added to bathwater

1.5 Comparison with Previous Work

This book covers 57 medical conditions organized into seven areas, the largest area being cancer which includes 16 types. A total of 31 cannabis compounds are investigated. The web supplement to this book includes approximately 1,400 references. Three other books contain similar material.

Backes's *Cannabis Pharmacy* is a comprehensive treatment of medical cannabis. Part 3 lists 50 cannabis strains, giving detailed information on each. Of particular note is the mention of each strain's key cannabis compounds. This type of information is essential for choosing varieties for specific medical conditions. Part 4 lists 50 medical conditions and provides a detailed readout on how THC and CBD help each condition. Part 4 cites 637 references.

Part 2 of Holland's *The Pot Book* discusses the potential harms and risks associated with cannabis. It covers roughly the same ground as Chapter 6 of this book. Chapters 24-28 and 37 discuss fifteen topics in-depth, with an emphasis on physical pain. CBD, THC, and synthetic cannabinoids are investigated. These chapters cite 280 references.

Frye's *The Medical Marijuana Guide* covers a wide range of topics, but its main overlap with this book comes in Chapter 5, which covers the use of CBD and THC in treating 40 severe medical conditions. Chapter 5 cites 101 references.

1.6 The Online Web Supplement to this Book

A web supplement includes 1,400 references that substantiate claims made in this book. Interested readers may obtain guest access to the supplement as follows: Go to <u>hempforhealth.net/cannabis/</u>, press the cancel button, and follow the instructions.

In the web supplement, mousing over a given citation (†) produces a popup reference that links directly to a representation of the corresponding work. Here is an example:

are designed to handle a specific medical condition. However, work along these lines has begun†.

Aside from ch... *Pharmacological Foundations of Cannabis* ...d
consuming in... *Chemovars [Project Description]*. Abstract. Lewis ...d
THCA, several ... M, Russo E, Smith K. Planta Medica. Online
Traditionally, (... November 21, 2017. ...re
are water-solu... ...ble
and digests faster than a tincture. Several techniques for creating powders are in use, but the common element is to create a powder

As in this example, each of the referenced works has an online presence. In most cases, the referenced online presence consists of an abstract or the full text of the referenced work.

2: Arthritis

THC and CBD help control arthritis symptoms, which is well known. These and 15 other cannabis compounds, mainly cannabis terpenes, may deter arthritis progression. The 15 are:

α-humulene
β-caryophyllene
apigenin
β-pinene
d-limonene
geraniol
eucalyptol
β-eudesmol
α-terpineol
eucalyptol
trans-nerolidol
β-caryophyllene oxide
α-pinene
4-terpineol
α-terpinene

Fourteen of these are terpenes, the exception being the flavonoid apigenin. *Appendix A: Common Cannabis Compounds* provides a brief introduction to these compounds.

The traditional approach to consuming terpenes is through aromatherapy — the inhalation and topical absorption of essential oils. Aromatherapy is a well-known approach to the treatment of arthritis pain. The new element reported here is its potential use in retarding the progression of arthritis.

A discussion of salient characteristics of common kinds of arthritis provides the basis for identifying cannabis compounds that, based on animal studies, may slow the progression of arthritis.

2.1 Types of Arthritis

Arthritis is a chronic inflammation of joints. According to the Arthritis Foundation, there are more than 100 different forms of arthritis, including osteoarthritis, rheumatoid arthritis, spinal arthritis, and psoriatic arthritis.

Osteoarthritis, the most common form, is traditionally viewed as a degenerative disease caused by wear and tear. However, obesity leads to a higher prevalence of osteoarthritis in non-weight-bearing areas as well as weight-bearing areas. Inflammatory cytokines are found in arthritic joints, contributing to arthritis progression. Moreover, inflammatory cytokine levels increase with age. So, there is reason to believe that inflammation either causes or strongly contributes to osteoarthritis.

Elevated levels of TNF-α, IL-1, and IL-6 occur in osteoarthritis — in the synovial fluid that lubricates the joints, in the membranes that hold the synovial fluid, and in the bone below a joint's cartilage. The link with obesity is that fat tissue is a source of inflammatory cytokines.

Increasing age brings increasing levels of inflammatory and erosive chemicals throughout the body, some of which are secreted by aging cartilage. There is increased systemic inflammation, increased inflammation of the joints, and increased chemically induced deterioration of cartilage.

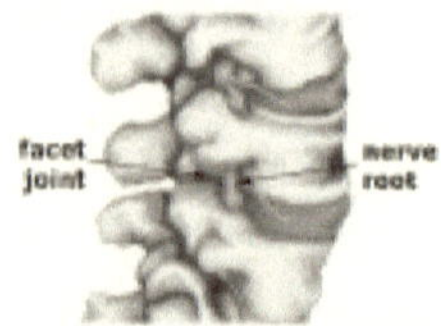

Spinal arthritis is usually a form of osteoarthritis. It occurs most commonly in the lower back or neck. Again, inflammation plays a key role. Spinal arthritis is associated with inflammation and degeneration of the vertebrae, facet joints, and disks, as illustrated in the above image. The degeneration leads to a narrowing (stenosis) of the spinal canal. The result is pressure on nerves leaving the spine that initially causes back pain and muscle spasms. The pinched nerves may include those associated with the lower extremities, causing pain to radiate downward through the pelvis, buttocks, legs, and knees. The pinched nerves may also cause bladder problems, including urgency and frequency of urination.

Ankylosing Spondylitis is an inflammatory arthritis of the spine. There is evidence that a particular bacterium can cause this form of arthritis. In this case, the cannabis compounds guaiol, BCPO (β-caryophyllene oxide), linalool, eucalyptol, and α-terpineol may help kill the bacterium.

The implicated bacterium is Klebsiella pneumoniae. The effectiveness of guaiol, caryophyllene oxide, linalool, eucalyptol, and α-terpineol was determined by studying traditional Australian herbal remedies, specifically, Tasmanian mountain pepperberry.

Rheumatoid arthritis is an autoimmune disease. The immune system attacks the synovial membranes that hold the fluid that lubricates the joints. Psoriatic arthritis is also an autoimmune disease. Its first symptom is usually psoriasis. With both conditions, pain is lessened, and disease progression is slowed by suppressing inflammation.

2.2 Fighting Arthritis

In a survey of Canadian cannabis users, the most popular strains for arthritis were Sweet Skunk CBD, OG Shark, Cannatonic, and CBD House Blend. Sweet Skunk CBD is a high-CBD strain whose primary terpenes include α-pinene, β-myrcene, and trans-nerolidol.

A 2018 paper presenting the research on Canadian cannabis preferences includes an outstanding review of previous relevant research. It concludes that their survey presents the first published research to explicitly address the fact that different strains have different medical benefits. The information on Sweet Skunk CBD comes from the Leafy website. The presence of trans-nerolidol in Sweet Skunk CBD is somewhat unusual.

CBD appears to reduce arthritis pain and deter joint damage. Moderate doses of CBD have proved more effective than large or small doses. THC also has an anti-inflammatory effect and has been shown to reduce pain and slow cartilage erosion. The terpene α-pinene has deterred the breakdown of cartilage and may also deter arthritis progression.

CBD and THC have both reduced pain and inflammation and have prevented nerve damage in animal models of osteoarthritis. A clinical trial demonstrated a significant analgesic effect of the Sativex brand of THC+CBD in rheumatoid arthritis. The use of CBD brought improvement in an animal model of arthritis used to study rheumatoid and reactive arthritis. One motivation for using THC is that it tends to be less toxic than the commonly used low-dose methotrexate. THC stimulates the CB2 cannabinoid receptor, which is more highly expressed in rheumatoid arthritis than in osteoarthritis.

The CB2 agonist JWH-133 has reduced inflammation and bone destruction in a mouse model of arthritis, and the same may be true of the stronger CB2 agonist β-caryophyllene (BCP).

The anti-inflammatory and anti-catabolic effects of d-limonene and α-pinene in human cartilage cells have been observed.

Arthritic pain and inflammation appear to be primarily caused by the four inflammatory cytokines IL-1, IL-6, TNF-α, and IL-17. These cytokines promote the initiation and progression of common forms of arthritis, including osteoarthritis, rheumatoid arthritis, septic arthritis, and post-traumatic arthritis. Much of the destruction is performed through IL-1 stimulation of nitric oxide production. An additional source of inflammation and destruction occurs when new blood vessels invade cartilage; healthy cartilage does not contain blood vessels.

For each destructive mechanism, the presentation proceeds in four steps: cannabis compounds that help, the mechanism's causal role in arthritis, conventional medicines whose success may block that mechanism, and, finally, an explanation of how the identified cannabis compounds block the destructive mechanism.

In some cases, there is a lack of research on lowering cytokines that have been elevated by arthritis. In these cases, it has been necessary to substitute educated guesses based on research into lowering cytokines that have been raised in other diseases such as cancer or rat paw edema. The same problem concerns research on preventing blood vessels from invading cartilage.

The IL-1 Cytokine

CBD, THC, BCP (β-Caryophyllene), α-humulene, geraniol, trans-nerolidol, d-limonene, α-terpineol, eucalyptol, and 4-terpineol may retard the progression of arthritis and associated pain by lowering IL-1 levels.

Causal Link. People living with arthritis, including those with post-traumatic arthritis, have high levels of IL-1α, IL-1β, TNF-α, and IL-17. These cytokines contribute to bone loss by stimulating the production of *osteoclasts*—cells that break down cartilage. IL-1α, IFN-γ, and TNF-α all induce apoptosis (programmed cell death) in bovine cartilage. This finding is relevant to most forms of arthritis, including osteoarthritis, rheumatoid arthritis, psoriatic arthritis, and ankylosing spondylitis.

Conventional Treatments. Multiple studies have shown that blocking IL-1 helps. The human body already has an IL-1 antagonist that lowers

IL-1, and there is a synthetic analog, anakinra (brand name Kineret), that lowers IL-1 levels and slows the progression of rheumatoid arthritis. Moreover, the body has a 'decoy' receptor that binds nitric oxide non-productively to IL-1, again blocking its inflammatory role and helping in an animal model of arthritis. Since blocking IL-1 helps, it may also be the case that lowering IL-1 helps.

Cannabis Compounds. THC lowered IL-1β in a brief human trial and in an animal model of RA. Both CBD and THC lowered IL-1β in chemically stressed mouse microglial cells. CBD lowered IL1-β and TNF-α in a mouse model of multiple sclerosis. BCP (β-caryophyllene) lowered IL-1β and TNF-α in in vitro tests.

Nerolidol inhibited IL1-β and TNF-α in mouse peritonitis. Perillyl alcohol reduced IL-1β and TNF-α in a rat model of stroke, and eucalyptol lowered IL-1.

α-Humulene lowered IL-1β and TNF-α in rat paw edema. Geraniol lowered IL-1β and TNF-α in rat tongue cancer. Perillyl alcohol, a metabolite of d-limonene, lowered IL-6, IL-1β, and TNF-α in a rat model of stroke.

The IL-6 Cytokine

CBD, THC, BCP, d-limonene, α-terpineol, 4-terpineol, eucalyptol, and apigenin may retard the progression of arthritis and associated pain by lowering IL-6 levels.

Causal Link. People with osteoarthritis or rheumatoid arthritis have elevated IL-6, which is thought to play an active role in disease progression and increased pain.

Conventional Treatments. The drug tocilizumab lowers RA disease activity by blocking the IL-6 receptor. The experimental drug sarilumab lowered RA disease activity by lowering IL-6 levels directly, but it failed to win FDA approval due to some fatalities. These results suggest that other ways of lowering IL-6 may help as well.

Cannabis Compounds. CBD lowered IL-6 in ischemic rat hearts and in chemically stressed mouse microglial cells. THC lowered IL-6 in a brief human trial and in an animal model of rheumatoid arthritis. THC also reduced IL-6 in chemically stressed macrophages and in an eternalized mouse microglial cell line. BCP lowered IL-6, IL-1β, and TNF-α in an immortalized microglia cell line used to study neuroinflammation.

Perillyl alcohol, a metabolite of d-limonene, lowered IL-6, IL-1β, and TNF-α in a rat model of stroke. α-Terpineol lowered IL-6 in human cheek cells stressed with desiccated orange juice. α-Terpineol and 4-terpineol (aka terpinen-4-ol) lowered both IL-6 and IL-1β in chemically stressed human macrophages. Eucalyptol lowered IL-6, IL-1β, and TNF-α in various in vitro and animal models of inflammation. The flavonoid apigenin lowered IL-6 in chemically stressed mice.

The TNF-α Cytokine

CBD, THC, BCP, eucalyptol, geraniol, α-humulene, α-terpineol, and apigenin may retard the progression of arthritis and associated pain by lowering TNF-α levels.

Causal Link. TNF-α is implicated in destroying bone and cartilage in osteoarthritis and post-traumatic arthritis.

Conventional Treatments. The commercial TNF-α inhibitors adalimumab (Humira) and infliximab (Remicade) bind directly to TNF-α, thereby disabling it. They have demonstrated effectiveness in treating rheumatoid and psoriatic arthritis as well as psoriasis itself. Inflammatory hand osteoarthritis has been successfully treated by blocking TNF-α with the off-label use of etanercept (Enbrel, Benepali). The success of TNF-α blocking drugs suggests that lowering TNF-α via cannabis compounds may help in the same way.

Cannabis Compounds. As noted above, CBD, BCP, nerolidol, perillyl alcohol, α-humulene, eucalyptol, α-terpineol, and geraniol all lower TNF-α. THC also lowered TNF-α in an animal model of rheumatoid arthritis

The flavonoid apigenin lowered TNF-α in an experimental model of mouse pancreatitis. Apigenin lowered TNF-α and upregulated the anti-inflammatory cytokine IL-10 in mouse leukemia macrophages.

The IL-17 Cytokine

BCP, CBD, and THC may be of benefit in rheumatoid arthritis by slowing bone loss and lowering IL-17 levels.

Causal Link. The breaking down of bone tissue is a normal part of bone metabolism. This process is carried out by specialized bone cells called osteoclasts. In rheumatoid arthritis, there are too many osteoclasts. Here's what happens: IL-23 induces synovial tissue to produce IL-17, which promotes the production of new osteoclasts. These cause synovial inflammation, cartilage and bone degradation, and joint destruction, according to in vitro and animal experiments. Much of this chaos is also apparent in ankylosing spondylitis.

Conventional Treatments. Secukinumab and ixekizumab (IL-17 neutralizing agents), and perhaps brodalumab (IL-17 receptor antagonist), have shown promise in treating psoriasis, psoriatic arthritis, and rheumatoid arthritis.

Cannabis Compounds. CBD lowered IL-17 in animal studies. THC lowered IL-17 in an in vitro study. The CB2 agonist JWH-133 lowered

IL-17 in macrophages, so the same is likely to be true of the stronger CB2 agonist BCP.

Nitric Oxide

α-Humulene, α-terpinene, α-pinene, β-pinene, and d-limonene may help with arthritis by lowering nitric oxide levels.

Causal Link. Nitric oxide is produced in cartilage due to stimulation by IL-1 and, for rheumatoid arthritis, TNF-α as well. Nitric oxide directly stimulates the destruction of cartilage in osteoarthritis, inflammatory arthritis, and especially rheumatoid arthritis.

Conventional Treatments. Reducing nitric oxide has reduced inflammation and inhibited cell death in cartilage and synovial membrane.

Cannabis Compounds. It may also be the case that nitric oxide-suppressing cannabis compounds impede arthritis progression. α-Humulene, α-terpinene,

α-pinene, and β-pinene have lowered nitric oxide levels. d-Limonene has reduced nitric oxide indirectly by inhibiting IL-1β.

Blood Vessel Invasion of Cartilage

CBD, THC, BCP, BCPO, d-Limonene, and β-eudesmol may help with arthritis by preventing inappropriate angiogenesis in which new blood vessels invade cartilage.

Causal Link. The destruction of cartilage by nitric oxide and other factors is followed by new blood vessels invading cartilage. This abnormal angiogenesis occurs in several types of arthritis, including osteoarthritis, rheumatoid arthritis, and chronic septic arthritis. It is stimulated by inflammation, at least in the case of osteoarthritis. In the case of rheumatoid arthritis, angiogenesis leads to the growth of "pannus" tissue that covers the synovial membrane and releases additional chemicals that destroy cartilage, bone, tendons, ligaments, and blood vessels.

Conventional Treatments. There have been some successes in treating arthritis by inhibiting angiogenesis. In rheumatoid arthritis, blockade of TNF-α and IL-1 significantly inhibits VEGF. This key signaling protein promotes the growth of new blood vessels. Szekanecz and Koch have enumerated several more angiogenesis inhibitors.

Cannabis Compounds. Although there has been no research on slowing angiogenesis in cartilage with cannabis compounds, there have been some results on slowing angiogenesis in cancer. CBD in colon cancer and glioblastoma; THC in breast cancer and glioblastoma; BCP viz JWH-133 in glioma; BCPO in breast and prostate cancer; β-eudesmol in cervical, gastric, and liver cancers; and d-limonene

in gastric cancer.

3: Pain

Research has shown that cannabis compounds can help with physical pain and chemotherapy-induced nausea. A report from the National Academies of Sciences, Engineering, and Medicine has provided carefully worded support.

This chapter explores the kinds of physical pain that cannabis compounds help alleviate. Altogether, 16 cannabis compounds are relevant. *Appendix A: Common Cannabis Compounds* introduces these compounds.

Typical physical pain is triggered by pain receptors in the skin, muscles, joints, etc. Neuropathic pain originates within the nervous system. Psychological pain comes from painful thoughts, feelings, and emotions. Both psychological pain and neuropathic pain can masquerade as typical physical pain.

This chapter discusses typical physical pain, neuropathic pain, cancer pain, and dysfunctional mystery pain. Mystery pain includes fibromyalgia, migraines, and adverse reactions to HPV vaccinations.

The exposition is organized as a series of explanations. Each explanation ends with a door that opens onto a summary of supporting research. The supporting research contains *dagger citations*. Mousing over a dagger brings up its corresponding reference hyperlinked to the supporting research.

3.1 Typical Physical Pain

Typical pain is a response to damaging or potentially damaging physical stimulation. Technically, typical pain is called nociceptive pain, and pain receptors are called nociceptors.

Typical pain is often caused by inflammation, which is a local response to cellular injury that initiates the elimination of noxious agents or damaged tissue. In this case, the first line of defense is usually to use anti-inflammatory compounds. An alternative to anti-inflammatories is to block the perception of pain. Other options include yoga, stretching exercises, and meditation.

Inflammation

Inflammation-fighting medications include NSAIDs such as aspirin and ibuprofen, the COX-2 inhibitor celecoxib (Celebrex), steroids such as hydrocortisone and prednisone, and cannabis compounds.

CBD, CBDA, THCA, CBC, and THCV are anti-inflammatory and may reduce sensitivity to pain. THC is anti-inflammatory at moderate doses but may be inflammatory at high doses. THC together with CBD or CBDA may work better than either one alone because THC works differently.

BCPO (β-Caryophyllene oxide) is comparable to aspirin in strength. It acts both locally as an anti-inflammatory and centrally as a pain-perception blocker. Unlike commercially produced NSAIDS, BCPO actively protects rather than erodes stomach linings.

α-Humulene, eucalyptol, linalool, and α-bisabolol are anti-inflammatory and pain-relieving. α-Bisabolol is known to act synergistically with the commercial NSAID diclofenac. These conclusions are based on animal studies.

Pain Perception

Pain perception blocking can occur in several ways:

- Block the activation of pain receptors.
- Block its propagation up the spinal cord.

- Block pain perception within the brain.

Pain blockers may also be able to send signals down the spinal cord that stop upward-moving pain signals. Opioids, NSAIDs, and several cannabinoids, including CBD and CBC, can block pain this last way. The best-known pain blocker, acetaminophen, appears to block pain both in the brain and in the spinal cord.

THC and morphine are synergistic in mice. BCP attenuates acute pain and acts as a local anesthetic, blocking pain perception at its source. Linalool has reduced typical nociceptive pain in animal studies. It blocks pain at the top of the spinal cord.

3.2 Neuropathic Pain

Unlike typical nociceptive pain, neuropathic pain originates within the pain-sensing and reporting nerves themselves. Such pain may be constant or sporadic. It may seem either localized or diffuse. Two notable cases are damaged nerves and severed nerves. Chronic nerve irritation is a form of nerve damage.

Damaged Nerves

Inhalation of marijuana is effective for neuropathic pain in HIV as well as central and peripheral neuropathic pain. Raw hemp oil may help treat chronic nerve irritation. A combination of equal parts THC and CBD may dull painful neuropathic responses to normal stimulation. However, THC may not be effective for refractory neuropathic pain.

BCP (β-caryophyllene) is effective against neuropathic pain. Moreover, unlike opioids, it does not lead to tolerance. BCP is helpful for both recurrent and chronic pain. The addition of the omega-3 fatty acid DHA improves BCP's effectiveness. Eucalyptol also decreases neuropathic pain.

Severed Nerves

Marijuana may be helpful for some forms of post-operative pain. THC has reduced spasticity in patients with spinal cord injuries but was of only minor benefit for well-established trauma-induced pain. Neither marijuana nor THC alone or in combination with CBD may be helpful severed nerves. Examples include dental extractions, hysterectomies, and tears in the brachial plexus.

THC has helped with spasticity following spinal cord injuries.

A study testing marijuana on post-traumatic and postsurgical neuropathic pain got positive results, as did another study on postoperative pain that used a 2-to-1 preparation of THC and CBD.

However, even a high THC level was of only minor benefit for well-established trauma-induced neuropathic pain. Two studies that tested THC for postoperative and post-injury pain got negative results. Both found THC no better than a placebo. One study looked at dental extractions, and the other at hysterectomies. In another study, neither THC nor THC+CBD brought much relief from the pain of brachial plexus tears.

3.3 Cancer Pain

Established cancer treatments have many unfortunate, life-threatening side effects, including severe pain, nausea, vomiting, and dangerous, potentially irreversible weight loss. As explained below, several cannabis compounds can help. However, THC by itself may not be the most effective treatment. THC, even in conjunction with codeine, is only mildly effective at stopping cancer-related pain.

Chemotherapy Pain

CBD and BCP may help prevent peripheral neuropathy and resultant neuropathic pain caused by chemotherapy. In combination with THC, CBD can help with intractable pain not adequately treated with opioids. Some studies have found that THC was only effective at doses high enough to produce major side effects and is not associated with increases in lean body mass.

CBD with THC (Sativex, Nabiximols) reduces intractable cancer-related pain, including pain not adequately relieved by strong opioids, and it continues to be effective in long-term use. Animal studies suggest that CBD may effectively prevent chemotherapy-induced peripheral neuropathy. Co-administration of low doses of THC enhances its effectiveness. Animal studies also showed that BCP prevented peripheral neuropathy and resultant neuropathic pain caused by the chemotherapy drug paclitaxel.

Nausea and Vomiting

Nausea is a diffuse sense of unease typically perceived as an urge to vomit. The compounds CBDA and THCA in raw marijuana flowers control nausea more effectively than CBD and THC, respectively. Δ^8-THC has been highly effective in controlling vomiting associated with conventional chemotherapy in children. Δ^8-THC is well suited to this use, as it is less intoxicating than Δ^9-THC

THC itself appears to work differently from conventional therapies and is often helpful for vomiting in cases where conventional drugs fail. It can be used as a monotherapy but may be more effective when combined with conventional drugs. The addition of CBD also makes THC more effective.

Δ^8-THC has been effective in controlling vomiting in children. Δ^9-THC was better in children than metoclopramide syrup and prochlorperazine tablets.

CBDA displays significantly higher potency at inhibiting nausea and vomiting than CBD. THCA appears to be more potent than THC. THC itself seems to work differently and is often helpful for vomiting in cases where conventional drugs fail.

Comparing THC with other therapies, the following appears to be the case:

- THC is less effective than levonantradol, a synthetic cannabinoid, in terms of nausea reduction and unwanted side effects.
- THC is comparable to prochlorperazine, thiethylperazine, and metoclopramide in reducing nausea and vomiting.
- THC appears to be more effective than cyclophosphamide, fluorouracil, and doxorubicin hydrochloride.
- THC improves the performance of methotrexate, but not Adriamycin or Cytoxan.
- THC, combined with CBD given as an adjunct to standard therapies, is better for nausea and vomiting than standard therapies alone.

Cachexia/Anorexia

About half of all patients with advanced cancer experience cachexia, an involuntary severe weight loss accompanied by muscle wasting. It seriously lessens the quality of life. It is associated with poorer outcomes. It is generally not reversible by increasing caloric intake. Treatment is challenging. Cachexia is not the same as anorexia, which is weight loss driven by an overpowering desire to be thin.

Low-dose THC may bring modest weight gain for several reasons. THC improves appetite. It also enhances the senses of smell and taste that cancer can destroy. Patients have also reported improved mood and reduction of pain. However, despite these perceived benefits, taking THC for nausea has not inspired significant enthusiasm. Rats given CBG (cannabigerol) or CBN (cannabinol) ate more food and ate more frequently. CBD is generally thought to promote weight loss.

Megestrol acetate appears to be superior to THC in terms of increased appetite and weight gain. Moreover, adding THC to megestrol acetate provides no additional benefit.

Ghrelin and THC do some of the same things, but ghrelin has some additional properties that may be useful for treating cachexia. It inhibits protein breakdown in patients with cancer cachexia, and it has anti-inflammatory, anti-apoptotic, and anxiolytic effects.

In an animal study, CBG and CBN stimulated weight gain, whereas CBD was associated with weight loss. CBG and CBN are known to have few side effects. But so far, they have been tested only on animals.

The many clinical practice articles and systematic reviews—and systematic reviews of systematic reviews—illustrate the challenging nature of treating cancer-related cachexia.

The evidence for THC's ability to promote weight gain is modest at best. In a small-scale study, low-dose THC brought minor weight gain. However, a phase III clinical trial failed to show that THC increases weight. The evidence for increased appetite is more robust. Patients have reported improved appetite and a heightened sense of smell and taste. As an aside, marijuana and obesity are also inversely correlated despite the fact that marijuana gives people the munchies.

In small-scale studies, cachexia patients taking THC have reported improved mood, better sleep, and more relaxation. They have also experienced a reduction in pain and fatigue. These results are consistent with a study of anorexic women without cancer. However, a clinical trial failed to observe these benefits.

In one study, cachexia patients received low-dose orally administered THC augmented with a small amount of CBD. Most patients dropped out. A well-designed clinical trial also failed to generate enthusiasm.

In a small-scale study, dronabinol, a form of THC, proved to be inferior to megestrol acetate. Adding Megestrol acetate to THC provided no additional benefit.

THC shares some significant properties with ghrelin, another compound being investigated for the treatment of cachexia. They are both agonists for not only the CB1 receptor but the ghrelin receptor as well. However, ghrelin has some additional attractive properties. It inhibits protein breakdown in catabolic conditions such as cancer cachexia. It has anti-inflammatory, anti-apoptotic, and anxiolytic effects as well

Rats given CBG (cannabigerol) or CBN (cannabinol) ate more food and ate more frequently.

3.4 Dysfunctional Mystery Pain

Researchers often refer to pain that they cannot explain in terms of an apparent stimulus or causal damage to the nervous system as "dysfunctional pain." Current examples of dysfunctional pain include fibromyalgia, irritable bowel syndrome, interstitial cystitis, migraines, and intractable pain following HPV vaccinations.

Fibromyalgia

Fibromyalgia is a medical condition defined by the presence of chronic widespread pain, fatigue, waking unrefreshed, cognitive symptoms, lower abdominal pain or cramps, and depression. Patients who smoke marijuana have seen significant improvement, especially in reducing pain and stiffness. Two consumer-oriented articles speak highly of high-CBD strains for fibromyalgia.

Migraines

Migraine is a disorder characterized by recurrent moderate to severe headaches. Researchers know a lot about migraines — the various kinds of migraines, how the primary triggers work, and many of the genes involved. Yet the exact cause remains a mystery, and commercially recommended treatments are not always effective. England's National healthcare service, the American Migraine Foundation, and Wikipedia all support the view that the causes of migraines remain unknown.

A survey of two thousand Canadian medical marijuana users found common traits among the most popular strains for taming migraine headaches. They were strains whose chemical makeup was very high in THC/THCA but low in CBD/CBDA. They were also low in β-caryophyllene and the sedative β-myrcene. Research suggests that marijuana decreases the frequency of migraine headaches.

The Canadian results about migraines are from a 2018 survey that established that different strains of marijuana have different medical benefits. Observational studies confirm the benefits of using marijuana both for decreased frequency of migraines and for reducing opioid dependence.

HPV Vaccinations

Intractable pain following HPV vaccinations is thought to be caused by a malfunction of the autonomic nervous system. Treatment with

CBD-enriched hemp oil has resulted in significantly reduced body pain.

3.5 Concluding Thoughts on Pain

A survey of 2,897 patient self-reports from an online cannabis community indicated that 97% could reduce opioid use while taking cannabis, and 81% felt that cannabis by itself was more effective than taking cannabis with opioids. A prospective study of 2,736 elderly patients at a specialized medical cannabis clinic where patients received customized treatments got similar results. Almost all patients reported improvement, with an average drop in pain score from 8 to 4 on a scale of 0 to 10.

These studies suggest that patients who play a significant role in managing pain tend to have better outcomes than in studies where all choices are in the hands of those performing the study.

In addition to comparing the relative amount of pain relief obtained from various cannabis compounds, it may be helpful to consider the relative risks involved. More than 47,000 people died from opioid overdoses in 2018. A few thousand died from adverse NSAID side effects the same year. There has been no reported overdose death from smoked marijuana. Moreover, very few deaths have resulted from marijuana-induced complications to other illnesses.

Given these statistics, we should ask whether patients in pain prefer risking death from conventional pain medications to risking pain from potentially ineffective cannabis compounds. But patients are often not allowed to choose between cannabis and prescription pain killers. Why? Financial incentives are likely involved. In 2015, Americans consumed 80% of the world's opioids at a cost of $19 billion. The tobacco and alcohol industries have also lobbied against marijuana legalization.

As of this writing, cannabis is still a Schedule 1 drug, meaning that it has no established medical benefit. This perspective has strongly influenced coverage of cannabis in the popular press.

4: Neurological Conditions

This chapter addresses the following neurological conditions: cognitive decline, Alzheimer's disease, multiple sclerosis, atrophic lateral sclerosis, Parkinson's disease, Huntington's disease, epilepsy, glaucoma, restless leg syndrome, and hot flashes. Strokes are covered in Chapter 7: Cardiovascular Conditions[1].

4.1 Cognitive Decline

Cognitive impairment occurs in approximately 36% of adults age 71 and older. Of these, roughly 14% are classified as having dementia. However, dementia prevalence increases with age, reaching 37% among individuals aged 90 and older. These percentages vary somewhat from one study to the next. The relevance of cannabis compounds for treating impairment does not appear to be strongly influenced by the degree of impairment.

Several general strategies are available for fighting cognitive decline. Neurogenesis is possible in some cases.

General Strategies

Some of the best approaches to preventing neurodegeneration don't involve cannabis compounds. Avoiding environmental neurotoxins helps. The starting point is knowing what they are and how to avoid them. Reviewing a list of *environmental neurotoxins* may help.

Toxin removal is also essential, but the most effective removal technique may be a deep, dreamless sleep. During sleep, the need for oxygen subsides, then blood volume drops and makes way for waves of cerebrospinal fluid to enter and wash away the toxins, including

---

1. http://pagenotes.com/cannabis/cardiovascular.htm#stroke

amyloid-beta. Unfortunately, modern people tend to suffer from insomnia. Little is known about whether sleep aids, including those listed in the Sleep Disorders discussion in Chapter 5: Psychiatric Conditions, interfere with the wash cycle.

A third general strategy is to neutralize toxins instead of removing them. CBD has been found superior to both alpha-tocopherol and Vitamin C in protecting neurons of the rat cerebral cortex from toxicity. Finally, there is the possibility of supporting the brain's microglial cells. These cells are found throughout the brain and spinal cord. They eat damaged neurons, cellular debris, foreign substances, microbes, and cancer cells, among other things. BCP (β-caryophyllene), CBD, and THC can protect microglial cells by suppressing inflammation.

A fourth strategy that works in some parts of the nervous system is neurogenesis — the process of adding new nerve cells to the nervous system.

Several degenerative neurological conditions involve prions — misfolded proteins capable of replication. They cause Creutzfeldt–Jakob disease and are implicated in several other illnesses such as amyotrophic lateral sclerosis (ALS), Alzheimer's disease, Parkinson's disease, and Huntington's disease, not to mention animal spongiform encephalopathies. They spread from cell to cell and throughout the brain. In animal studies, CBD has been shown to prevent prion accumulation and protect neurons against prion toxicity.

Promoting Neurogenesis

Hope for reversing neurodegeneration in adults rests partly with the three areas of the brain that are capable of neurogenesis. One area, dubbed the "SVZ," produces neurons that travel to the olfactory bulb, where they process smells. The second area is within the hippocampus, which is responsible for forming new long-term memories and many other things. The third area is the striatum, which processes reward stimuli and performs stimulus-response learning.

Either acute or chronic administration of high-dose CBD has restored damaged memory in mice, possibly through neurogenesis in the hippocampus. CBD also enhanced neurogenesis in the hippocampus of young adult mice, as did CBC.

A chronic low dose of THC restored cognitive function in old mice, apparently due to restored hippocampal function. However, higher doses of pure THC may not be suitable because THC induces temporary memory impairment in humans, whereas THC+CBD does not. BCP (β-caryophyllene) may stimulate neurogenesis in older mice and humans. An animal study showed that the CB2 agonist JWH-133 promoted neurogenesis. BCP is a more potent CB2 agonist than JWH-133, so BCP may as well.

The significance of these results in restoring hippocampal function is that, on the one hand, the hippocampus is essential to the formation of new memories. On the other, it is easily damaged by stress, Alzheimer's disease, and mental illnesses, including depression, schizophrenia, and PTSD. Patients with mild but observable cognitive impairment a have 10-15% loss of hippocampus volume, those with early Alzheimer's have a 15-30% loss, and in those with moderate Alzheimer's, it may reach 50%.

4.2 Alzheimer's Disease

Alzheimer's disease is a progressive form of presenile dementia characterized by impaired memory which is followed by impaired thought and speech and finally complete helplessness.

Roughly 70% of those with dementia have Alzheimer's dementia. Of the remaining categories, 17% have vascular dementia, and 13% have some other form—in decreasing order, an undetermined form, Parkinson's dementia, normal-pressure hydrocephalus, frontal lobe dementia, alcoholic dementia, traumatic brain injury, and Lewy body dementia.

Alzheimer's has understandably attracted more research interest than other types of dementia. This interest is true of research into cannabis compounds for dementia as well. While humans are the only animals that can get Alzheimer's, transgenic mice with human Alzheimer's genes have been developed. They provide some insights but do not fully replicate Alzheimer's.

This section starts with a brief introduction to Alzheimer's, followed by research related to controlling damage from amyloid-beta and tau, and lastly, controlling behavioral symptoms.

Alzheimer's Overview

Alzheimer's develops both inside and outside of brain neurons. Inside, the tau protein, which is involved in constructing and maintaining a cell's cytoskeleton, becomes damaged. Damaged tau then forms clumps known as neurofibrillary tangles that interfere with normal cell function.

Outside, amyloid-beta proteins (Aβ proteins) become misfolded and form clumps known as plaques that are toxic to neurons. Aβ itself is an intermediary waste product formed during the metabolism of a normal protein. Unfortunately, forming plaques thwarts the successful disposal of Aβ, setting up a vicious cycle. Crucially, Aβ damages tau.

In the brain's learning and memory centers, the neurotransmitter acetylcholine plays an essential role in forming and preserving memories by binding to several types of acetylcholine receptors. Unfortunately, Aβ can disable and destroy some types of acetylcholine receptors.

The brain's acetylcholine is mainly produced by neurons in the basal forebrain and then distributed throughout the brain and central nervous system. Unfortunately, Aβ can kill the acetylcholine-producing neurons, reducing acetylcholine levels by as much as 90%.

Neurons dispose of used acetylcholine using the acetylcholinesterase enzyme. Acetylcholinesterase inhibitors can raise acetylcholine levels, providing symptomatic relief. Unfortunately, this does nothing to slow the progression of the disease.

As is usually the case with brain damage, dying neurons release free radicals, causing inflammation and collateral damage.

Minimizing Amyloid Beta's Damage

In vitro studies show that low-dose THC reduces inflammation, is effective at lowering Aβ levels, and inhibits Aβ aggregation. The cannabinoids THC and CBN act synergistically to remove intraneuronal Aβ, reduce oxidative damage, and protect neurons from loss of energy. An in vitro study suggests that CBD reduces Aβ-induced toxicity.

BCP (β-Caryophyllene) can reduce Aβ plaques.

Apigenin dissolves Aβ and thus inhibits neuron death. Apigenin also protects the capillaries that maintain the blood-brain barrier, thereby preventing Aβ from robbing neurons of their blood supply.

Linalool protects against Aβ-induced cognitive deficits and damage.

An in vitro experiment suggests that CBD inhibits Aβ-induced damage to tau protein. CBD Reduces Aβ-Induced neuroinflammation and promotes hippocampal neurogenesis. CBD lowers toxicity caused by Aβ.

Eucalyptol also mitigates Inflammation caused by Aβ deposits. β-Caryophyllene inhibits neuroinflammation as well.

Linalool restores cognitive and emotional functions via an anti-inflammatory effect.

Controlling Behavioral Symptoms

In a mouse model of the early stages of late-onset Alzheimer's, CBD+THC preserved memory and reduced learning impairment. CBD and THC had the same effect individually but were less effective.

Both mice and humans make and recognize social contacts. Both Alzheimer's and a mouse model of Alzheimer's destroy this capability. In the mouse model, long-term treatment with CBD preserved the capacity to recognize social contacts.

THC is an acetylcholinesterase inhibiter, meaning that THC also provides symptomatic relief. It inhibits Aβ aggregation more effectively than some commercial acetylcholinesterase inhibitors. α-pinene is a potent acetylcholinesterase inhibitor and is anti-inflammatory as well.

4.3 Multiple Sclerosis

Multiple sclerosis is an autoimmune inflammatory disease that wreaks havoc by stripping protective insulation, known as myelin, from the surfaces of neurons in the brain and spinal cord.

A consensus of medical experts is that using equal parts of CBD and THC improves patient-reported spasticity symptoms.

Inhibiting Progression

CBD was neuroprotective in a mouse model of MS. It lowered the inflammatory cytokine IL-17, thereby reducing inflammation.

CBD provides long-lasting protection against the harmful effects of inflammation in a viral model of multiple sclerosis. It strengthens the blood-brain barrier and inhibits the pro-inflammatory cytokine IL-1β.

One experimental model of multiple sclerosis is experimental autoimmune encephalomyelitis; CBD is effective in this model. So are CBG and BCP.

THC suppressed immune response in a mouse model of multiple sclerosis; the significance is that multiple sclerosis is believed to be an autoimmune disease.

Symptom Relief

THC has been helpful for muscle immobility. Whole cannabis extracts have also helped.

THC and whole cannabis extracts have been helpful with urge incontinence. THC, in combination with CBD, has also effectively reduced urinary incontinence.

THC in combination with CBD effectively treats insomnia, neuropathic pain, and other neurological symptoms of multiple sclerosis.

A spray preparation of CBD+THC (Sativex) directed towards the mucous surfaces of the mouth is helpful for multiple sclerosis symptoms, including neuropathic pain, dysesthesia, allodynia, spasticity, muscle spasms, and sleep disturbances.

A small anonymous survey of 112 cannabis smokers with multiple sclerosis rated the effectiveness of street cannabis against common symptoms. The results, in decreasing order of benefit, were: spasticity, chronic pain of extremities, acute paroxysmal phenomenon, tremor, emotional dysfunction, anorexia/weight loss, fatigue states, double vision, sexual dysfunction, bowel, and bladder dysfunctions, vision dimness, dysfunctions of walking and balance, and memory loss. Spasticity was improved for 92% of the patients, whereas memory loss was improved for only 30%.

A CBG metabolite alleviated neuroinflammation in an animal model of MS.

4.4 Parkinson's Disease

Parkinson's disease results from the die-off of dopamine-producing neurons that supply parts of the brain involved in movement and reward, specifically, the substantia nigra.

BCP (β-Caryophyllene) protects against oxidative stress, neuroinflammation, and the destruction of dopaminergic neurons in the substantia nigra. The positive impact of BCP may be related to the reduction of CB2 receptors.

THCV provides symptom relief and protects against loss of neurons in the substantia nigra. THC, THCA, and CBD are all protective of dopamine-producing neurons in vitro. Most of the beneficial effects of these cannabis compounds appear to be from their value as antioxidants.

CBD significantly reduced Parkinson-related psychosis in half a dozen outpatients. CBD improved excessive physical movement during the rapid-eye phase of sleep.

As a negative result, an orally administered cannabis extract showed no objective or subjective improvement in dyskinesias or parkinsonism. Nor did smoked marijuana. But in one study, cannabis did help with Parkinson's involuntary muscle movements.

4.5 Essential Tremor

Essential tremor is about ten times as common as Parkinson's. It involves shaking of hands and other extremities and is thought to be caused by a loss of fine motor control in the cerebellum. The cerebellum plays a central role in fine motor coordination and is involved in many forms of cognition. Essential tremor is consistently associated with cognitive impairment and, in older people, dementia.

Some credible personal stories about the benefits of CBD for essential tremor have been posted in various places, including one on a Mayo Clinic site and several in the closed Facebook group "Essential Tremor on CBD."

Recently, a team at the University of California at San Diego has gone forward with a clinical trial based on personal stories and positive results for similar diseases such as Parkinson's. The trial uses a 20:1 CBD:THC product imported from Canada.

4.6 Huntington's Disease

Huntington's is an inherited genetic illness that causes premature death of brain neurons in the striatum, which coordinates movement, and in the frontal cortex, which controls thinking and emotions. This is the disease that killed Woody Guthrie.

Conventional treatments provide symptomatic relief: physical therapy and tetrabenazine for movement problems; antidepressants, mood stabilizers, and atypical antipsychotics for psychiatric symptoms.

β-Caryophyllene and similar chemicals may protect against neuron injury and reduce neuroinflammation.

CBG has shown significant neuroprotection in animal models of Huntington's disease.

CBD has shown neuroprotection in animal models, apparently due solely to its antioxidant properties. However, in human clinical trials, CBD by itself appears to be neither helpful nor harmful. CBD+THC is neuroprotective and delays disease progression. However, THC by itself seems to be counterproductive.

4.7 Traumatic Brain Injury (TBI)

TBI Patients who tested positive for THC when admitted to a Level 1 trauma center had a 2.4% mortality rate. In contrast, patients who tested negative had an 11.5% mortality rate. After adjusting for age and other confounding factors, those with THC still did better. This improvement could be partially due to the lowering of the TNF-α Cytokine.

In one case of severe TBI, a combination of CBD and essential fatty acids accompanied dramatic recovery.

Several research articles report that CB2 receptor agonists help with brain injury. The same is likely true of the natural CB2 receptor agonist BCP. However, the newer synthetic CB2 agonists are progressively more potent, so adequate dose sizes could be significantly different.

Hypoxia in newborn infants. Newborns often suffer from oxygen deprivation during delivery. The traditional treatment is hypothermia, administered as soon after birth as possible. It is somewhat effective. Pure CBD administered intravenously to (human) newborns was also somewhat effective, but the two treatments combined have produced the most robust results.

The use of CBD alone in newborn mice allowed quantitative measurement of improvement. Surprisingly, the therapeutic effect was seen when treatment was delayed by as much as 18 hours.

4.8 Epilepsy, Seizures, Convulsions

Epilepsy is a group of non-communicable neurological disorders characterized by recurrent epileptic seizures — periods of unusual behavior, sensations and sometimes loss of awareness.

Available evidence supports the adjunctive use of CBD for epilepsy as accepted medical practice. Much of the progress in this area is due to Charlotte Figi's success with Dravet syndrome. Cannabidiol has performed well in several clinical trials — Dravet syndrome, Sturge-Weber syndrome, Lennox-Gastaut, and other forms of treatment-resistant epilepsy.

BCP inhibited seizures and protected against associated neurological damage in mouse experiments. These results may be due mainly to BCP's anti-inflammatory properties.

An animal study suggests that THCV may be useful for treating epilepsy. Another study indicates that Linalool may compare favorably with diazepam and phenytoin.

4.9 Restless Leg Syndrome

Restless Leg syndrome provides a recent example of how cannabis research progresses. A few desperate people experiment — with CBD, for instance. Then they get good results and post emphatic personal stories in odd places. Somewhere in the world, a doctor becomes intrigued and enlists colleagues to do some case studies. With good results, they recommend clinical trials.

4.10 Glaucoma, Other Eye Conditions

Interest in cannabinoids for eye problems began with the observation that smoked marijuana and several individual cannabinoids can temporarily reduce intra-optic eye pressure. Marijuana may also have a neuroprotective effect in reducing the damage caused by glaucoma.

Research suggests that cannabinoids such as CBD and THC can play a direct role in slowing disease progression. Such diseases include glaucoma, diabetic retinopathy, age-related macular degeneration, and retinitis pigmentosa.

Before light can reach an eye's rods and cones, it travels through several other layers of neurons. The first is the "wires" that carry information to the optic nerve. Here is a quick summary of what's known, gleaned from a review of the research and a sample research paper.

The retina layers are packed with cannabinoid-sensitive receptors — the cannabinoid receptors CB1 and CB2 plus four others: GPR55, TRPV1, PPARα, and PPARγ. Why would the retina be so heavily involved in cannabinoid metabolism? Endocannabinoids play a key role in protecting the retina from neurotoxins produced during retinal neurons' normal functioning.

Boosting endocannabinoid levels has decreased neurotoxic damage associated with glaucoma and a few other diseases. In a few animal studies, THC and CBD have also slowed disease progression.

In an animal study, chronic topical administration of either CBG or CBD significantly reduced intra-ocular eye pressure, but CBD had undesirable side effects. THC, delta 8-THC, CBN, and CBG all reduce intraocular pressure.

In a clinical trial, inhaled THC reduced both blood pressure and intraocular eye pressure for 3 to 4 hours. Both of these effects were greater in subjects with hypertension.

Cannabinoids are oils, and eyes are mostly water. CBD applied to the outside of an eye isn't readily absorbed. Overcoming this problem is an active area of research. Options include water-miscible cannabinoid suspensions and water-soluble procannabinoids with cannabinoid metabolites.

4.11 Hot Flashes

Hot flashes involve feelings of intense heat with sweating and a rapid heartbeat. Each occurrence typically lasts from 2 to 30 minutes. Moderate to severe hot flashes continue after menopause for nearly five years on average but continue for ten years or more in a third of post-menopausal women.

Hot flashes involve a dysregulation of the brain's temperature control mechanism in the hypothalamus. It regulates core body temperatures between an upper threshold for sweating and a lower threshold for shivering. There is a *thermoneutral* zone within which the body regulates temperature without resort to sweating or shivering.

Hot flashes are associated with narrowing the thermoneutral zone coupled with the core body temperature going above the upper threshold. Among women who do not have hot flashes, the thermoneutral zone is approximately 0.72 °F. In contrast, it is virtually nonexistent among women with hot flashes. High brain levels of the norepinephrine neurotransmitter shrink the thermoneutral zone. So does activation of the sympathetic nervous system, which is the portion of the autonomic nervous system responsible for the fight-or-flight response. The hypothalamus controls the autonomic nervous system.

The drug clonidine lowers norepinephrine release, raises the sweating threshold, and reduces shivering, thus reducing hot flashes. The hormone estradiol, the FDA-approved approach to hot flashes, raises the sweating threshold and lowers norepinephrine levels. A third strategy for lowering hot flashes is to go directly after the sympathetic nervous system. Slow, deep breathing calms the sympathetic nervous system and brings a 50% reduction in hot flashes (practice required).

Finally, we come to how cannabis compounds can reduce hot flashes. To begin with, it seems they can, judging from women's emphatic personal stories.

There has been no systematic research on how cannabis compounds affect hot flashes. However, from the above, it appears that beneficial cannabis compounds calm the sympathetic nervous system, reduce norepinephrine levels, and lower central body temperature. THC lowers central body temperature. THC may also inhibit norepinephrine in sympathetic nerves.

Many indica marijuana strains contain the sedative terpene d-linalool; it depresses the autonomic nervous system and may thus also widen the thermoneutral zone.

5: Psychiatric Conditions

This chapter is mainly organized according to the American Psychiatric Association's *Diagnostic and Statistical Manual of Mental Disorders*. However, chemical addictions are treated separately in Chapter 6: Chemical Addictions. Psychiatric consequences of neurological conditions are also treated separately in Chapter 4: Neurological Conditions.

5.1 Neurodevelopment

Fragile-X syndrome

Fragile X syndrome is caused by an inherrited genetic defect in a gene that protects against mental retardation. Studies show that CBD helps with fragile-X symptoms. It helps with social avoidance and anxiety. It also improves sleep, feeding, motor coordination, language skills, anxiety, and sensory processing.

Autism Spectrum Disorder

Autism spectrum disorder affects how people interact with others, communicate, learn, and behave. Symptoms appear within the first two years of life.

Small-scale studies of autistic children found that cannabis extracts with a very high CBD/THC ratio usually improved autistic symptoms without undue intoxication. The symptoms that improved included

- attention deficit/hyperactivity disorder.
- depression.
- restlessness, rage attacks, and other behavioral disorders.
- tics and other motor deficits.

- autonomy deficits.
- communication and social interaction deficits.
- cognitive deficits.
- seizures.
- sleep disorders.

Tourette Syndrome

Tourette Syndrome is a condition of the nervous system that causes people to have involuntary tics — sudden twitches, movements, or sounds that they do repeatedly.

THC has successfully treated Tourette syndrome. A single dose was adequate. THC treatments continued to be effective over six weeks. The effects persisted for several weeks after treatment was stopped. THC successfully treated a refractory case as well.

5.2 Schizophrenia

Schizophrenia involves three kinds of problems:

- positive symptoms - experiencing what's not there
- negative symptoms - not experiencing what is there
- cognitive symptoms - thinking problems

Negative symptoms are more challenging to treat than positive symptoms.

Detailed Definition. The identified symptoms of schizophrenia vary somewhat from one source to the next. The following list is typical.

Positive Symptoms

- hallucinations
- delusions

- disorganized speech and thinking

Negative Symptoms

- blunted emotional response
- blank facial expression
- dull voice
- trouble experiencing happiness
- social withdrawal
- loss of libido
- apathy

Cognitive Symptoms

- poor executive function
- trouble paying attention
- working memory deficits
- lack of self-awareness

Executive function involves translating ideas into decisions and actions. Self-awareness includes awareness of being schizophrenic.

The above list of schizophrenia symptoms draws from lists given by the Mayo Clinic, Living with Schizophrenia, and Wikipedia.

Schizophrenia is one illness where THC is strongly contraindicated. Daily use of high-THC street marijuana triples the chance of developing schizophrenia. Those who do develop schizophrenia do so several years sooner. Moreover, even in those without schizophrenia, marijuana often stimulates schizophrenia-like symptoms. These warnings do not apply to balanced preparations containing equal amounts of THC and CBD.

CBD is at least as effective in treating schizophrenia as conventional antipsychotics. Clozapine is better at treating symptoms but is typically used only for treatment-resistant patients due to its side effects.

Patients with treatment-resistant schizophrenia may not respond to CBD. Its use as a supplement to other antipsychotics may not help.

Several studies have reported the effect of marijuana on non-psychotic users. Regular users of high THC / low CBD marijuana had significantly increased psychotic symptoms compared to non-users and users of balanced THC/CBD preparations. CBD was able to block positive symptoms, especially delusions and hallucinations. These effects are visible in functional MRI scans. CBD affected the same regions as THC, but with opposite changes, even in non-users. But for non-users, these changes in brain function did not affect behavior.

Daily use of high-THC street marijuana tripled the chances of developing schizophrenia compared to non-users. A related observation is that marijuana use in early adulthood predicts higher use, later on, of prescription antipsychotics, mood stabilizers, and antidepressants. For those who smoke street marijuana and do develop psychosis, the age of onset is three years sooner. However, marijuana use versus non-use does not predict what symptoms will later develop in those who develop schizophrenia.

As a supplemental therapy, CBD often improves positive symptoms of schizophrenia. This result is seen both in clinicians' reports and standardized tests. CBD was comparable to the antipsychotic amisulpride in a clinical trial for treating both positive and negative symptoms. The likely reason is that CBD raised anandamide levels. Amisulpride and thus CBD compare favorably with most conventional antipsychotics. Only clozapine is better at treating symptoms, but its side effects are such that it is reserved for treatment-resistant patients.

CBD is no magic bullet. In two studies, patients with treatment-resistant schizophrenia failed to respond to CBD monotherapy. There was also a clinical trial where adjunctive use of CBD was unable to help with cognitive symptoms of schizophrenia.

There is a genetic link between heavy cannabis use and developing schizophrenia. So drawing cause-and-effect conclusions about the relationship between the two conditions requires caution.

The above research differs significantly from research on cannabis compounds in treating other illnesses. The more informative studies regarding schizophrenia have all been on humans rather than animals. And the only two cannabis compounds studied have been THC and CBD. Why?

5.3 Bipolar Disorder

Bipolar disorder is a mood disorder characterized by periods of depression and periods of abnormally-elevated energy or happiness.

Cannabis use is strongly correlated with bipolar disorder. According to a lengthy research review, it is associated with an early age of onset, increased severity, increased disability, increased risk for suicide, increased risk of manic symptoms, and general disability. None of the studies reviewed address the issue of cause and effect, and there is good reason for suspicion. People with bipolar disorder are seven times more likely to use cannabis than others. One possibility is that THC has a causal role in the development of bipolar disorder. But a competing explanation based on patient reports is that people with bipolar disorder are attracted too marijuana because its calming effect tends to smooth out bipolar highs and lows.

One small-scale study found that marijuana may bring about a "substantial decrease in a composite measure of mood symptoms."

Moreover, marijuana does not cause cognitive impairment beyond that already due to bipolar disorder. Furthermore, cannabis use has been associated with a lower remission rate following successful treatment for bipolar.

Unfortunately, none of this bipolar research involves a clear intention to treat, and none of it has moved beyond the study of undifferentiated street marijuana.

5.4 Depression

Depression is a mental and behavioral disorder characterized by loss of interest or a loss of feeling of pleasure in activities that usually bring joy to people.

Smoking marijuana reduces depression. The best strains for depression are those high in CBD and low in THC. A couple of puffs may be enough to produce significant relief. Animal studies provide additional results on depression.

CBD lessens depression by stimulating serotonin receptors in the brain. Thus, CBD substitutes for serotonin in the same way that THC substitutes for anandamide. Moreover, CBD is rapid-acting. Moderate doses of THC have antidepressant properties, whereas high doses do not.

CBC also has antidepressant properties, as does BCP (β-caryophyllene). The terpenes linalool and d-limonene also have antidepressant effects. Their mechanism of action is different from that of THC or CBD.

Unhappiness. People with consistently high levels of the endocannabinoid anandamide tend to be happier and thus less depressed. The cannabinoids CBD, CBN, and THC all raise anandamide levels.

Two large-scale surveys showed that marijuana reduces objective measures of depression. One of the surveys dealt with Canadian medical marijuana users who used the Strainprint app. This utility provides exact data on marijuana strains. That survey showed that high-CBD, low-THC strains worked best. Surprisingly, two puffs sufficed to cut depression levels in half. The apparent explanation behind CBD's antidepressant properties is that it is a 5-HT1A serotonin agonist.

CBD's effectiveness is similar to imipramine, but unlike imipramine, CBD acts quickly. THC, CBD, and CBC all have antidepressant effects in animal models of despair.

BCP has antidepressant effects because it is a CB2 agonist. Perhaps THC's antidepressant effect is also due to its being a CB2 agonist. The mechanisms behind the antidepressant effects of linalool and limonene are different from those of cannabinoids.

Mouse experiments have shown that CBD, CBN, and THC inhibit the breakdown of anandamide. Higher levels of anandamide are statistically associated with greater happiness. In more detail, worldwide surveys have shown that happiness is related to a gene variant that slows anandamide's breakdown.

5.5 Anxiety, Stress, Panic

These are similar conditions:

- Anxiety: Inner turmoil and feelings of dread over anticipated events.
- Stress: Psychological pain involving feelings of strain and

pressure.
- Panic: Sudden overpowering fright and extreme anxiety.

Marijuana strains that have a balanced content of CBD and THC may be the best for stress and anxiety, anxiety more so than stress.

CBD has been found helpful for social anxiety disorder and anxiety induced by public speaking. However, CBD may not be helpful for anxiety that is not caused by anxiety-producing events. Moderate doses of CBD are more effective than large doses.

Low doses of THC may provide modest relief in stressful encounters, while high doses are counterproductive. THC itself is known to induce anxiety. CBD can counter such anxiety, which is yet another reason to avoid CBD deficient strains of marijuana.

Linalool and linalyl acetate are the principal components of lavender. Lavender's effectiveness as an antidepressant may be comparable to the benzodiazepine lorazepam (Ativan). Of course, lavender is superior to benzodiazepines in side effects, including freedom from addiction. Lavender is also useful for restlessness and insomnia. Eucalyptol, apigenin, and d-limonene may also reduce anxiety.

A large-scale survey of medical cannabis users found that marijuana strains with a balanced CBD and THC content are best for stress and anxiety. Alleviation from stress may require as many as ten puffs. The survey relied on the Strainprint app to obtain exact data on what products users consume.

Patients with anxiety or sleep disorders were given CBD over three months in a large case series and showed improvement. CBD noticeably reduced anxiety in teens with a social anxiety disorder. In a similar experiment, patients with a social anxiety disorder were almost normal after taking CBD. One study of normal subjects found CBD ineffective for general anxiety but effective for anxiety induced by simulated public speaking. Another study found that moderate doses of CBD, but not large doses, quelled anxiety caused by public speaking.

Using functional MRI imagining on humans, it is possible to observe, in real-time, CBD blocking anxiety as it travels from the amygdala to the anterior cingulate gyrus.

Inhaling eucalyptol may reduce anxiety before surgery. The flavonoid apigenin reduced stress in animal studies, and the terpene d-limonene reduced anxiety.

5.6 Post Traumatic Stress Disorder (PTSD)

PTSD is characterized by residual feelings of stress or fright experienced even when one is no longer in danger. It is a frequent result of trauma. Roughly 17% of the veterans from Iraq and Afghanistan have PTSD. Data from a New Mexico shows that taking marijuana for PTSD can result in a 75% reduction in symptoms.

In a survey of two thousand medical cannabis users, the most popular strains for PTSD were Jack Herer, Island Sweet Skunk, White Widow, and Jean Guy. Jack Herer is a relatively high THC strain whose top terpenes include pinene, myrcene, and trans-nerolidol.

Rats tend to get PTSD from hanging out with hungry house cats. Happily, repeated CBD administration prevents them from having long-lasting trauma-induced anxiety. The same is true of traumatized humans. For example, a traumatized ten-year-old girl responded to CBD after prescription medications had failed.

According to a Veterans Health Administration report, roughly 17% of the veterans from Iraq and Afghanistan have PTSD. A survey of medical marijuana use for PTSD in New Mexico found that marijuana use results in a 75% reduction in symptoms. New Mexico was the first state to approve marijuana for PTSD.

In a survey of two thousand medical cannabis users, the most popular strains for PTSD were Jack Herer, Island Sweet Skunk, White Widow, and Jean Guy. The most common forms of ingestion were smoking and vaporizing (vaping). The paper presenting this survey includes an outstanding review of previous relevant research. This 2018 survey was the first research to address the undeniable fact that different strains have different medical benefits.

Rats that received repeated CBD administration starting an hour after a cat encounter avoided long-lasting trauma-induced anxiety. The same is true of traumatized humans. CBD acts to consolidate new fear-extinction learning. A 10-year-old girl who did not respond well to commercial medications and their adverse side effects maintained a decrease in anxiety and a steady improvement in the quality and quantity of sleep when given CBD.

THC appears to improve the effectiveness of fear-extinction training in which PTSD patients learn to calmly experience a traumatic memory that previously induced strong emotion. A 19-year-old male patient with a spectrum of severe PTSD symptoms discovered that some of his significant symptoms were dramatically reduced by smoking cannabis resin. His symptoms included intense flashbacks, panic attacks, and self-mutilation.

5.7 Sleep Disorders

Increased use of cannabis products is associated with decreased sales of OTC sleep aids. Multiple cannabis compounds have sedative properties.

In a survey of two thousand medical cannabis users, the most popular strains for insomnia were Lemon Sour Diesel, OG Shark, Skywalker OG, and Pink Kush. Lemon Sour Diesel has high THC and almost no CBD. Its top terpenes are caryophyllene, humulene, and linalool. THC induces sleepiness but brings impaired functioning and increased sleepiness the following day. CBD promotes improved sleep in insomniacs.

Among terpenes, linalool has sedative effects on mood states and the autonomic nervous system (which regulates heart rate, digestion, respiratory rate, pupillary response, urination, and sexual arousal). Animal studies have shown that d-Limonene, α-pinene, and terpinolene have sedative effects.

In Colorado, a month-by-month comparison of grocery store scanner data with month-by-month recreational cannabis access showed a shift from OTC sleep aids to cannabis as more cannabis dispensaries became available.

Among terpenes, linalool has sedative effects on mood states and the autonomic nervous system. In animal studies, d-Limonene had sedative and motor relaxant properties. For mice, the sedative effect of α-pinene is similar to that of Ambien. Terpinolene also has sedative effects.

5.8 Sex and Marijuana

People who smoke marijuana have more sex. Its use doesn't promote risky sexual behavior unless it is accompanied by heavy drinking. Marijuana increases overall satisfaction, sensitivity to touch, and the ability to relax during sex. But it may not increase desire, the intensity of orgasms, or the ease of achieving orgasms. There's a 10% chance that marijuana will actually make things worse.

Among teenagers, using marijuana may increase the likelihood of becoming sexually active and increase the possibility of having multiple partners.

Marijuana use is positively correlated with sexual frequency in men and women. Marijuana use does not increase the likelihood of risky sexual behavior unless accompanied by heavy drinking.

In a survey, a substantial majority said that marijuana increased overall satisfaction, sensitivity to touch, and the ability to relax during sex. Reports were divided on whether marijuana increased desire, the intensity of orgasms, or the ease of achieving orgasms. Reports also differed on whether marijuana helped with sex, but only 10% said it made sex worse.

Among teenagers, using marijuana may increase the likelihood of becoming sexually active. Among those who have had sex, it may increase the likelihood of having multiple partners. Among teenagers who occasionally play hooky and sometimes use marijuana, using marijuana while playing hooky on a given day increases the likelihood of having sex.

5.9 Concluding thoughts

A *psychoactive compound* is a chemical substance that changes brain function, resulting in alterations in perception, mood, consciousness, cognition, or behavior. Some psychoactive drugs have all five effects — sedatives, for example.

According to extensive, publicly available published research, the cannabis compounds listed in the following table appear to be psychoactive.

THC	Elevates mood, promotes sleep, reduces stress and anxiety, is an antidepressant, may be intoxicating, and may produce psychotic effects in large doses.
CBD	Prevents epileptic seizures, elevates mood, reduces anxiety, inhibits addiction relapse, fights schizophrenic psychosis, and is an antidepressant.
CBN	Elevates mood.
BCP	Elevates mood and helps with obsessive-compulsive disorder.
Linalool	Elevates mood, promotes sleep, lowers anxiety, is an anticonvulsant, and is an antidepressant.
d-Limonene	Reduces stress; is an antidepressant, sedative, and motor relaxant.
Terpinolene	Is a sedative and promotes sleep.

6: Chemical Addictions

The most common definition of *addiction* is that attempted cessation leads to the discovery that stopping is easier said than done. Further evidence of addiction is that use has caused problems severe enough to impair health, work, and personal relationships. Alcoholism, for example, shortens one's life span by 26 years on average. It causes one to miss work or be less productive, and it wreaks havoc with family life.

Published addiction rates are surprisingly speculative. They are typically given without reference to a definition of addiction and often equate usage rates with addiction rates. There has been research on how street marijuana affects chemical addictions but relatively little research on how specific cannabis compounds affect addictions.

The following sections cover tobacco, alcohol, opioids, cocaine, and marijuana addictions. The topics discussed include mortality, health effects, risk of addiction, and relationship to marijuana. Regarding mortality, the statistics apply to people living in the United States.

A final section addresses the impact of variations in the gene for the CB1 cannabinoid receptor that is responsible for the intoxicating effects of THC.

6.1 Nicotine and Tobacco

Mortality. Tobacco kills 1300 people a day.

Health Effects. Smokers are more prone to develop heart disease, stroke, and lung cancer. They are more prone to cardiovascular diseases, including strokes, heart attacks, and narrowing of blood vessels. COPD is more frequent and more severe in smokers, and the same goes for asthma. Smoking by either men or women adversely affects conception and pregnancy and increases congenital disabilities.

Risk of Addiction. There is widespread agreement that nicotine is the most addictive of the commonly used psychoactive drugs. The Nicotine addiction rate is around 32% of those who smoke regularly.

Relationship to Marijuana. Cannabis does contribute to the risk of tobacco addiction. Specifically, cannabis use is associated with increased initiation, persistence, and relapse to cigarette smoking. Moreover, tobacco addiction is predictive of marijuana addiction.

6.2 Alcohol

Mortality. Alcoholism kills 240 people a day.

Health Effects. The ill-effects include liver disease, heart disease, hypertension, stroke, and throat cancer.

Risk of Addiction. The American Psychiatric Association's DSM-5 uses the term Alcohol Use Disorder (AUD) rather than addiction. Briefly, AUD is an impaired ability to stop or control alcohol use despite adverse social, occupational, or health consequences. The rate of AUD is thought to be around 10% for men and 5% for women.

Relationship to Marijuana. Alcohol consumption increases the effects of THC by increasing THC levels. The terpene β-caryophyllene (BCP) and, even more so, β-Caryophyllene oxide (BCPO) may help with alcohol addiction by reducing alcohol consumption.

6.3 Heroin and Other Opioids

Mortality. Overdoses kill 130 people a day.

Health Effects. Long-term use damages the brain's white matter, causes increasingly severe addiction, and damages veins, nasal passages, or lungs depending on the route of administration. It also brings a continuing risk of overdose and death.

Risk of Addiction. Most opioids are less addictive than tobacco. Heroin, for example, has an addiction rate of perhaps 23% of those who use regularly.

Relationship to Marijuana. CBD may lessen the intensity of heroin relapse triggers. Methadone patients who regularly use marijuana tend to experience less severe heroin withdrawal symptoms during the initial methadone stabilization phase. However, marijuana use may not aid patients in opioid addiction treatment

6.4 Cocaine, Amphetamines

Mortality. Cocaine kills upwards of 40 people a day.

Health Effects. Long-term use damages the cardiovascular system and creates neurological damage. Cocaine, and more especially methamphetamine, damage the mouth, teeth, and nasal passages.

Risk of Addiction. It has an addiction rate of perhaps 17% of regular users.

Relation to Marijuana. Crack withdrawal symptoms are lessened by street marijuana. Jamaican women routinely use marijuana to minimize the undesirable effects of crack pipe smoking, specifically paranoia and weight loss. CBD and THC can help extinguish drug-motivated learned behavior in rats.

6.5 Marijuana

This section is about marijuana and marijuana-based products. The information reported here does not apply to synthetic marijuana products or flavored vape products. It also does not apply to flavored vape products. In some cases, the effects of marijuana may depend on the route of administration. For example, marijuana behaves differently depending on whether it is smoked or eaten.

Mortality. The conclusion of a 1973 animal study was that it is not possible to overdose on marijuana or even on THC.However, potentially fatal complications to existing conditions can result from marijuana use.

Risk of Addiction. Roughly 10% of regular marijuana users become addicted. Furthermore, roughly 30% have withdrawal symptoms when quitting. The total number of marijuana users who abuse marijuana or become dependent on it may be as high as 30%. There is evidence that marijuana addiction is easier to kick than alcohol addiction. However, marijuana is somewhat cross-addictive with other psychoactive substances.

People who begin using marijuana before age 18 are four to seven times more likely to become addicted than people who begin as adults.

Low, subclinical doses of THC have decreased marijuana craving and withdrawal symptoms. A clinical trial indicated that CBD reduces marijuana use.

Health Effects. Therapeutic doses appear to be safe and well-tolerated in adults, including older adults, whether healthy or frail or suffering from dementia. The following paragraphs discuss the possibility of harm to the brain, effect on the lungs, driving impairment, decrease in crime, and improved longevity.

Brain Development. Repeated high doses of THC may interfere with brain development, with long-term adverse consequences. The research results are not easily explained by other variables such as education, wealth, or the use of other drugs. These results are concerning because functional brain development continues until around age 25, and white matter development continues until middle age. However, one study shows that heavy marijuana use after age 18 is not associated with significant cognitive decline. The interference with brain development begins in utero.

In addition to overall brain development, there is the related issue of developing psychiatric problems. For most conditions, marijuana seems to help. The main exception is schizophrenia. See the schizophrenia discussion in Chapter 5: Psychiatric Conditions.

Effect on Lungs. Smoked marijuana does irritate the lungs and can cause chronic bronchitis. However, it does not significantly increase the risk of major illnesses such as emphysema or lung cancer. Moreover, the occasional use of marijuana may actually improve lung function.

Impact on Driving. The moderate use of marijuana does not affect crash risk when other variables such as alcohol use are accounted for. This finding is surprising because marijuana impairs neurocognitive performance and impairs driving lateral control. Possibly, drivers impaired by marijuana know they are impaired and drive accordingly.

Overall, legalization in Colorado has improved people's driving. It appears that when other factors such as the prevalence of drunk driving are factored in, marijuana is actually beneficial.

Impact on Longevity. Very little is know on how usage impacts longevity. It is known that marijuana has some adverse effects, such as increased periodontal disease and decreased bone mineral density. However, there are also some easily recognized positive indications.

Alcohol sales have dropped 12% In states with medical or recreational marijuana laws. Along with the decrease in alcohol sales, traffic fatalities have also declined.

Marijuana legalization has seen a shift away from the use of competing prescription drugs, something that is also likely to affect longevity. The shift is substantial in pain medications but is also significant for medications used to treat anxiety, nausea, seizures, and sleep disorders.

6.6 Genetic Influence

This section is rather technical, but it holds the key to who should and should not use THC. It sheds light on why people's responses to THC vary widely, with a few people having severe reactions.

Some of the genetic variation involves the CNR1 gene that codes for the CB1 cannabinoid receptor. That is the receptor responsible for the intoxicating effects of marijuana. Some involves the FAAH gene responsible for breaking down the endocannabinoid anandamide.

Briefly, locations within a gene with genetic variation are called SNPs (single nucleotide polymorphisms). Most SNPs come in pairs, one SNP from each of one's two parents. Typically, each SNP has a major common variant and a minor less common variant. The minor variant tends to be the more problematic of the two, with two copies more problematic than one. Technically, a SNP variant is an *allele*, and a SNP pair is a *genotype*. SNPs have somewhat random names of the

form rsxxxxxxx.

rs2023239

This SNP is on the gene that codes for the CB1 cannabinoid receptor. The minor rs2023239 allele is named C for cytosine. Possession of the C allele flies in the face of the nearly universal impression that marijuana has a mellowing effect. In a study published in 2019, C allele carriers who received THC experienced more anger and hostility than those who received a placebo.

Those with the C allele also experience stronger cravings while using marijuana and have greater withdrawal symptoms in response to abstinence.

A study of patients with alcohol dependence linked the minor C allele with greater subjective reward from alcohol as well as greater alcohol consumption

rs324420

This SNP is on the gene that codes for the FAAH enzyme, which breaks down anandamide. The minor rs324420 allele is named A for adenine. It results in less of the FAAH enzyme, causing higher anandamide levels. Anandamide is correlated with happiness. Unfortunately, the minor A allele also carries an increased risk for substance use disorder.

7: Cardiovascular Conditions

Studies of the overall cardiovascular impact of smoked marijuana have been inconsistent. Some suggest a benefit, while others suggest the opposite. However, CBD and other specific compounds show promise.

The following topics outline the various kinds of cardiovascular impairment: hypertension, dyslipidemia, atherosclerosis, myocardial ischemia, myocarditis, heart failure, ischemic strokes, and heart attacks.

7.1 Hypertension

In human studies, CBD reduced blood pressure, and the results were more pronounced in people who had high blood pressure to begin with. Prolonged THC use lowered blood pressure and heart rate; these results are from a 1975 study. Eucalyptol has lowered blood pressure in rats.

7.2 Dyslipidemia

Dyslipidemia involves abnormal blood levels of lipids — such as cholesterol and triglycerides. It can involve HDL levels that are too low or LDL levels that ae too high. The primary concern is with LDL levels.

Cholesterol-lowering alternatives to statins are of interest because statins block a primary metabolic pathway. They block not only cholesterol but 30,000 other molecules, including heme, vitamin K, coenzyme Q10, and all steroid hormones.

Linalool and eucalyptol synergistically inhibit the production of cholesterol in a manner competitive with statins, judging from their effect on liver cells. Camphene is comparable to lovastatin in its ability to lower cholesterol in rats. THCV and CBD may also be useful as they reduce lipid levels in liver and fat cells. These results are significant in that they reduce the incidence of fatty liver disease and help avoid obesity.

While LDL cholesterol has been tied to cardiovascular problems, oxidized LDL is a much stronger predictor of coronary heart disease. LDL particles risk cardiovascular disease when they enter blood vessel walls and become oxidized. In an in vitro study, terpinolene and γ-terpinene inhibited oxidation of LDL cholesterol.

7.3 Atherosclerosis

Atherosclerosis is a buildup of abnormal fatty deposits and fibrous tissue in the inner layer of the arteries. In a word, clogged arteries.

Treatment with the terpene β-caryophyllene reduces cardiac lipid content and improves the antioxidant/oxidant ratio in heart tissue of hypercholesterolemic rats. Low-dose oral THC reduces the progression of atherosclerosis in mice via a role similar to that of β-caryophyllene.

7.4 Myocardial Ischemia

CBD is of substantial benefit in myocardial ischemia (reduced blood flow to the heart), and it reduces associated ventricular arrhythmias. β-Caryophyllene may also be of value due to its anti-inflammatory and antioxidant properties. These results are based on animal and cellular studies.

7.5 Myocarditis

CBD may reduce myocarditis, which is inflammation of the heart muscle.

7.6 Heart Failure

Heart failure occurs when the heart cannot pump sufficiently to maintain blood flow to meet the body's needs. The condition is associated with poor tolerance to exercise. IL-1β makes the condition worse. In mice, blocking IL-1β brings improvement. As noted in *Appendix B: Taming Cytokines[1]*, CBD, β-caryophyllene, nerolidol, d-limonene, eucalyptol, d-humulene, and geraniol all lower IL-1.

7.7 Ischemic Stroke

Ischemic strokes reduce blood flow to the brain and are often triggered by blood clots. The reduced blood flow kills neurons, and dying neurons kill more neurons. CBD can reduce this cascade of dying neuros, but only at moderate doses. It increases cerebral flow and reduces cell death in the area of the stroke. CBD provides potent, long-lasting neuroprotection in mice, whether administered before or after an induced stroke. The protection is mainly due to CBD's anti-inflammatory properties.

After an ischemic stroke, the blood-brain barrier is weakened by a lack of glucose and oxygen, thus allowing an influx of substances toxic to the brain. CBD inhibits this weakening of the blood-brain barrier.

In animal studies, preventive treatment with CBD was effective, and repeated treatment after the stroke continued to be effective without developing tolerance. Treatment with β-caryophyllene before a stroke decreased swelling, brain damage, and mitochondrial dysfunction after the stroke.

Perillyl alcohol, a metabolite of the terpene d-limonene, protected against cell death from reactive oxygen species after a stroke. Linalool was neuroprotective. α-Bisabolol was neuroprotective, probably due to

---

1. *http://pagenotes.com/cannabis/inflam-cytokines.htm*

its anti-inflammatory capability. Eucalyptol limited the damage after a stroke due to its anti-oxidative effect.

7.8 Heart Attack

A heart attack is a sudden blockage of blood flow to a part of the heart muscle.

Marijuana consumers are more likely to survive a heart attack.

IL-1β contributes to long-term damage after a heart attack, and blocking IL-1 limits damage. As noted above, CBD, β-caryophyllene, nerolidol, d-limonene, eucalyptol, d-humulene, and geraniol all lower IL-1.

α-Bisabolol protects heart muscle following a heart attack through its free-radical scavenging capabilities in rats.

8: Cancer

The research on cannabis and cancer dates back at least to 1974. Since then, human studies have repeatedly shown that a suitable combination of cannabis compounds and conventional methods such as chemo or radiation works better than either alone.

8.1 Cancer-Fighting Tasks

A bottom-up analysis of the research on cannabis and cancer identifies five different cancer-fighting tasks. These tasks are in addition to the well-known palliative task of treating cancer pain and nausea.

For example, one compound will inhibit invasion and metastasis, another turns off the ID1 oncogene, and a third kills cancer cells. How could they not be synergistic? These are examples of the entourage effect. Here are the five tasks.

1. *Killing Cancer Cells.* This can happen in two different ways.
    1a. In *apoptosis*, also known as *programmed cell death*, cells self-destruct.
    1b. In *necrosis*, they are killed by some outside force.
2. *Stopping Cell Replication.* This can also be done in a couple of ways.
    2a. *Cell-cycle arrest* prevents cells from reproducing.
    2b. *Angiogenesis* preventions' stops a tumor from growing new blood vessels.
3. *Inhibiting Invasion and Metastasis.* Tumors often try to evade defeat by creating new tumors in nearby locations (*invasion*) or distant locations (*metastasis*).
4. *Controlling Cytokines.* Inflammatory cytokines promote cancer growth, so it helps to lower these cytokines.

5. *Mutation Control.*
   5a. *Mutation deterrence* prevents mutation into new treatment-resistant forms.
   5b. *Genetic rep*air turns bad genes off and good genes on.

Types of Cancer

The following sections are listed in approximate order of decreasing death rate. In each section, the presentation is organized along the lines of the above five tasks. Some of the less deadly cancers are not well addressed by existing cannabis research.

8.2 Cancers of the Lung and Bronchial Tubes

Lung cancer causes the most deaths of any cancer, and the deadliest lung cancer is small-cell lung cancer. It has a survival rate of about 6%. It accounts for at most 15% of all lung cancers. The most common cancer is adenocarcinoma. It is a form of non-small-cell lung cancer that starts in the mucus glands that keep the lungs from drying out. Wikipedia has some details:

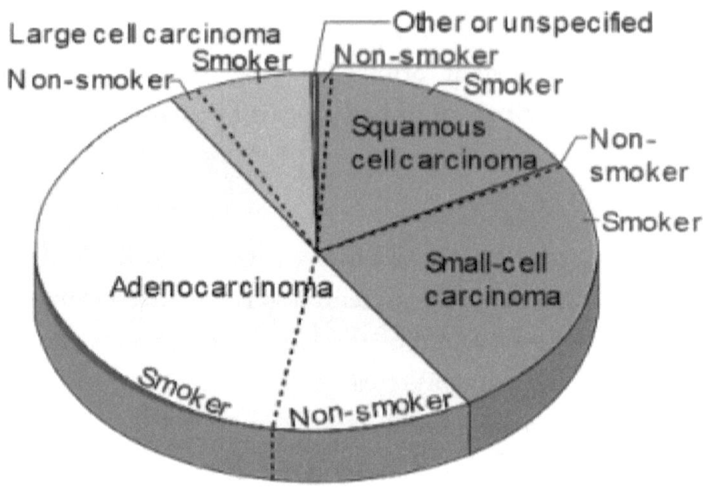

Killing Cancer Cells

Evidence about the effectiveness of cannabis compounds against small-cell lung cancer is sparse. However, there is a good deal of in vitro evidence regarding efficacy in killing adenocarcinoma and other non-small-cell cancer cells: CBD, α-humulene, BCPO (β-caryophyllene oxide), α-bisabolol, α-pinene, α-terpineol, d-limonene, and apigenin are all useful.

Finally, α-terpineol does inhibit small-cell lung cancer.

Stopping Cell Replication

The CB2 agonist JHW-133 inhibits angiogenesis, and, presumably, so does the stronger CB2 agonist BCP (β-caryophyllene).

Inhibiting Invasion and Metastasis

THC has been shown to inhibit invasion and metastasis in a xenograft model of lung cancer. In vitro studies have shown that CBD inhibits invasion of surrounding tissue.

Suppressing Inflammatory Cytokines

Elevation of the IL-1β cytokine is associated with a poor prognosis in patients with lung cancer. IL-6 stimulates tumor progression in non-small-cell lung cancer cells. IL-17 promotes tumorigenesis, angiogenesis, invasiveness, metastasis, and immune system tolerance. It inhibits apoptosis. IL-8 promotes angiogenesis in bronchial cancer.

Appendix B: Taming Cytokines has some general ideas on lowering inflammatory cytokines.

Controlling Gene Expression

α-Terpineol inhibits small-cell lung cancer by lowering genes that control transcription of DNA, cytokine production, and cell survival.

CBD significantly reduces the size and number of lung metastases by manipulating the Id1 gene.

8.3 Breast Cancer

Breast cancers are classified in various ways. *Ductal cancers* start in the milk ducts. *Lobular cancers* begin in the milk glands. *Invasive cancers* have spread to other parts of the breast. 70-80% of breast cancers are invasive ductal cancers. One also sees the term *adenocarcinoma*, referring to cancers that start in the epithelial cells lining the ducts and lobules. Breast cancer is the second most common cause of cancer death among women.

Invasive ductal carcinoma begins in a milk duct and then invades surrounding tissue. The cancer releases cells into the bloodstream, where the most aggressive survive to establish new metastatic tumors. In addition, the original tumor attracts circulating cancer cells in a self-seeding process. The tumor's attractants are IL-6 and IL-8.

Cancers that respond to estrogen are referred to as *HR-positive*. Cancers that respond to progesterone are *PR-positive*. Cancers that produce too much of the HER2 protein are *HER2 positive*. Cancers that meet none of these criteria are said to be *triple-negative*.

Virtually all of the research reported below consists of in vitro studies. It is suggestive of but not necessarily indicative of how cannabis compounds relate to human breast cancer.

Killing Cancer Cells

CBD induces apoptosis in triple-negative breast cancer cells. THC induces apoptosis of HER2-positive breast cancer cells.

α-Terpinolene is cytotoxic against adenocarcinoma cells. Linalool acts synergistically with the chemotherapy drug doxorubicin in fighting adenocarcinoma.

The cannabis flavonoid apigenin is cytotoxic against HER2-positive breast cancers. Apigenin is also effective against androgen-responsive human breast cancer cells.

BCPO (β-caryophyllene oxide) induces apoptosis in several kinds of breast cancer cells.

α-humulene, together with the chemotherapy drug paclitaxel, has exhibited significant cytotoxic activities against invasive ductal breast cancer cells, especially when combined with β-caryophyllene.

Stopping Cell Replication

THC inhibits cell cycle progression in cancerous breast epithelial cells. THC was able to impair tumor angiogenesis in a mouse model of HER2-positive breast cancer.

Inhibiting Invasion and Metastasis

CBD limits invasion and metastasis in adenocarcinoma cells. So does CBDA

Controlling Cytokines

Elevated IL-6 levels are generally associated with poor prognosis and low survival rates in patients with breast cancer. IL-6 is known to stimulate growth, invasion, and metastasis. IL-6 triggers signs of malignancy, both in human ductal breast cancer and in normal mammary glands. High levels of IL-1α and IL-6 are significantly correlated with a poor prognosis.

Elevated IL-1β directly promotes the invasiveness of triple-negative breast cancer cells. IL-1β induces IL-6 production and increases invasiveness and estrogen-independent growth in human breast cancer cells.

IL-22 promotes breast cancer, but the release of IL-22 is dependent on the release of IL-1β. IL-1β and IL-17 are implicated in breast cancer metastasis.

For general ideas on controlling cytokines, see *Appendix B: Taming Cytokines.*

Controlling Gene Expression

CBD turns off the ID1 oncogene in several types of breast cancer. CBDA lowers the COX2 gene as well as the ID1 gene. Both genes are overexpressed in invasive ductal carcinoma. THC limits progression by turning off the CDC2 gene.

8.4 Prostate Cancer

Although nonmetastatic prostate cancer now has a cure rate approaching 100%, prostate cancer is still the second leading cause of cancer death in men. In vitro studies suggest several cannabis compounds that may help.

Prostate cancer cells are classified as *androgen-dependent* if they need androgen and *androgen-independent* if they don't. Androgen-dependent cancers are often treated with androgen deprivation therapy, which works if they don't become androgen-independent.

Killing Cancer Cells

CBD has induced apoptosis in in vitro studies and reduced the size of androgen-dependent tumors in animal studies. THC is known to induce apoptosis of androgen-dependent prostate cancer cells.

BCPO (β-caryophyllene oxide) has induced apoptosis on several prostate cancer lines and is synergistic with the chemo drug doxorubicin. α-Humulene is cytotoxic against androgen-dependent prostate cancer cells.

The flavonoid apigenin promotes apoptosis and is synergistic with the chemo drug cisplatin.

Stopping Cell Replication

Menthol promotes cell cycle arrest in androgen-independent prostate cancer cells. The flavonoid apigenin accomplishes cell-cycle arrest and apoptosis in prostate cancer cells — both androgen-dependent and androgen-independent cells.

Inhibiting Invasion and Metastasis

BCPO inhibits invasion in prostate cancer cells. Menthol inhibits the motility of androgen-independent cancer cells.

Suppressing Inflammatory Cytokines

Patients with elevated levels of TNF-α and IL-1β have a poor prognosis. Elevated TGF-β is associated with angiogenesis, metastasis, and poor clinical outcome. IL-6 promotes prostate cancer.

CBD lowers IL-6 and IL-8 in several prostate cancer cell lines. See *Appendix B: Taming Cytokines* for general ideas on lowering cytokines.

Controlling Gene Expression

BCPO lowers gene expression to inhibit angiogenesis, cell proliferation, and metastasis.

8.5 Cancers of the Colon and Rectum

Roughly 95 percent of all colorectal cancers are *adenocarcinomas* — they start as polyps in the mucus glands of the colon or rectum and then become cancerous. Unless otherwise noted, the studies mentioned in this article were carried out on adenocarcinomas. They are primarily in vitro studies.

Colorectal cancer is the third leading cause of cancer deaths.

Killing Cancer Cells

CBD kills colon cancer cells. So does CBG. The following cannabis terpenes kill colorectal cancer cells: α-humulene, eucalyptol (aka 1, 8-cineole), borneol, and geraniol.

BCP (β-Caryophyllene) enhances the effectiveness of conventional cancer drugs when tested on chemo drugs such as paclitaxel and doxorubicin. β-Caryophyllene oxide, trans-nerolidol, and valencene also enhance the efficacy of doxorubicin. Geraniol enhances the effectiveness of the otherwise ineffective chemo drug 5-fluorouracil.

Stopping Cell Replication

A high-CBD cannabis extract reduced proliferation ib both in vitro and animal studies.

The following cannabis terpenes inhibit cell replication: BCP (β-caryophyllene), BCPO (β-caryophyllene oxide), geraniol, α-humulene, trans-nerolidol, valencene. Apigenin also inhibits replication.

Inhibiting Invasion and Metastasis

BCP (β-Caryophyllene) inhibits tumor motility, migration, and invasion in colorectal cancer.

Controlling Cytokines

THCA inhibits growth in colon cancer by lowering IL-8.

The inflammatory cytokines IL-1β, IL-6, IL-8, IL-17, IL-21, IL-22. TNF-α, and VEGF are all elevated in colorectal cancer. They all appear to promote cancer growth.

IL-8 stimulates the growth of human colon cancer cells. IL-1α promotes migration and angiogenesis. IL-8 and IL-17 promote invasiveness. IL-17 promotes metastasis. Most of these results are known to apply to colitis-associated cancers in particular.

Some general ideas on controlling cytokines are given in *Appendix B: Taming Cytokines*.

8.6 Pancreatic Cancer

Ethan Stewart survived metastatic neuroendocrine pancreatic cancer by using large quantities of whole cannabis extracts. His personal story begins with the question "Can Cannabis Cure My Cancer?" and ends with the observation: "My life is all the proof I need."

Killing Cancer Cells

THC and CBD induce apoptosis in pancreatic cancer cells. Perillyl alcohol and α-bisabolol are cytotoxic against pancreatic cancer.

Apigenin enhances the effectiveness of the chemotherapy drug gemcitabine in treating pancreatic cancer.

Cytokine Control

Elevated IL-1β predicts pancreatic cancer risk.

IL-6 is elevated in pancreatic cancer. It plays an essential role in the development of pancreatic ductal adenocarcinoma. However, IL-6 also stimulates insulin production in non-cancerous pancreas islets.

As noted in *Appendix B: Taming Cytokines*, CBD, THC, perillyl alcohol, α-Terpineol, 4-terpineol, eucalyptol, and apigenin may all help lower IL-6.

Inhibiting Invasion and Metastasis

BCP, α-Bisabolol, and Geraniol have an anti-proliferative effect against pancreatic cancer.

Apigenin enhances the anti-proliferative effect of chemotherapy drugs on human pancreatic cancer cells.

8.7 Cancers of the Cervix and Uterus

Killing Cancer Cells

BCPO (β-caryophyllene oxide) is cytotoxic against cervical cancer cells. BCPO has also improved the cytotoxicity of doxorubicin for cancer cells while decreasing its toxicity for normal cells.

Linalool is cytotoxic against cervical cancer cells. So are α-terpineol, eucalyptol, and 4-terpineol. The flavonoid apigenin induces apoptosis and cell cycle arrest against some forms of cervical cancer cells.

Preventing Angiogenesis

β-Eudesmol has inhibited angiogenesis in human cervical cancer cells.

Inhibiting Invasion and Metastasis

CBD inhibits invasion and metastasis in human cervical cancer. Apigenin inhibits the motility and invasiveness of cervical cancer cells

8.8 Cancers of the Liver and Bile Duct

Cancers of the liver are usually cancers of the liver tissues, as opposed to cancers of blood vessels or bile ducts within the liver. These are referred to as *hepatocellular carcinoma*. In addition, there are secondary cancers that originate elsewhere and metastasize to the liver.

Overexpression of the CB1 and CB2 cannabinoid receptors correlates with improved prognosis of patients with hepatocellular carcinoma. But stimulation of the CB1 receptor promotes cancer, suggesting that THC may be counterproductive.

Killing Cancer Cells

α-Pinene, linalool, β-caryophyllene oxide, α-terpineol, eucalyptol, 4-terpineol, α-pinene, d-limonene, and geraniol are all cytotoxic against hepatocellular carcinoma cells.

Halting Cell Division

α-Pinene and geraniol have inhibited cell division in human liver cancer.

Preventing Angiogenesis

β-Eudesmol inhibits the growth of new blood vessels.

Inhibiting Invasion and Metastasis

THC reduces the invasiveness of bile-duct cancer cells when administered at doses low enough to avoid killing the cancer cells.

Limiting Inflammatory Cytokines

IL-6 is overexpressed and contributes to tumor cell growth in bile duct cancer. See *Appendix B: Taming Cytokines*.

8.9 Leukemia

Leukemia generally refers to cancers of blood-forming tissues in the bone marrow. The disease usually affects one of the two major types of white blood cells: lymphocytes and granulocytes. Leukemias arising from lymphocytes are called lymphocytic leukemias; those arising from granulocytes are called myeloid or myelogenous leukemias.

Lymphocytic leukemia is composed of immature lymphocytes floating in the bloodstream. Immature lymphocytes are known as lymphoblasts, so lymphoblastic leukemia is another term for this type of leukemia. When lymphocytes mature, they leave the bloodstream and reside in the lymph system.

Lymphocytic cells are mainly B cells and T cells. Myeloid cells are primarily monocytes and macrophages.

In a clinical setting, both lymphocytic and myeloid leukemias can be classified as chronic or acute.

Human leukemias have significantly more CB2 receptors than other types of tumors. Surprisingly, CBD acts as an agonist for these CB2 receptors.

Unless otherwise noted, all studies are in vitro studies of human cells.

Lymphocytic Leukemia

Killing Cancer Cells

THC induces apoptosis in lymphocytic leukemia cells.

Eucalyptol kills leukemia cells. So does apigenin.

BCP and BCPO increase the effectiveness of the chemotherapy drug doxorubicin against doxorubicin-resistant childhood lymphoblastic leukemia cells.

α-Terpineol is cytotoxic against human lymphoblastic leukemia cells, chronic myeloid leukemia cells, acute myeloid leukemia cells, and acute erythroid leukemia cells.

4-Terpineol is cytotoxic against lymphoblastic leukemia T cells and human chronic myeloid leukemia cells. α-Bisabolol is cytotoxic against human B-chronic lymphocytic leukemia cells.

Myeloid Leukemias

Killing Cancer Cells

Linalool induces apoptosis in acute myeloid leukemia cells.

Chronic myeloid leukemia is usually the result of having the BCR-ABL gene. For these cancers, α-bisabolol dramatically enhances the chemotherapy drugs imatinib and nilotinib.

α-Terpineol is cytotoxic against chronic myeloid leukemia cells, acute myeloid leukemia cells, and acute erythroid leukemia cells. 4-Terpineol is cytotoxic against human chronic myeloid leukemia cells.

Terpinolene is cytotoxic against human myeloid leukemia cells. So is d-limonene. Eucalyptol is cytotoxic against myeloid leukemia cells as well as cancerous B cells.

Perillyl alcohol is effective in killing chronic myeloid leukemia cells.

Halting Cell Division

Apigenin induces cell cycle arrest in myeloid leukemia cells but also interferes with the commonly used chemotherapy drug vincristine.

Controlling Cytokines

IL-6 elevation contributes to the development of chronic myeloid leukemia.

Chronic myeloid leukemia patients have responded well to the IL-6 inhibitors dasatinib and imatinib. See *Appendix B: Taming Cytokines* for additional ideas on taming IL-6.

8.10 Lymphoma

Lymphoma takes the form of tumors in the lymph system that are made up of cancerous lymphocytes. Lymphoma differs from lymphocytic leukemia, which consists of immature cancerous lymphocytes floating in the bloodstream.

Killing Cancer Cells

CBD kills lymphoma cells.

Linalool is cytotoxic against human lymphoma cell lines. β-Caryophyllene and caryophyllene oxide induce apoptosis in human lymphoma cells. α-Pinene is cytotoxic against histiocytic lymphoma.

Halting Cell Division

d-Limonene inhibits the proliferation of murine lymphoma.

Controlling Cytokines

Elevated IL-10 plasma levels correlate with poor prognosis in patients with diffuse large B-cell lymphoma.

IL-10 provides resistance to cytotoxic drugs in Non-Hodgkin's Lymphoma by blocking apoptosis.

IL-1α and IL-8 immunoreactivity are increased in patients with cutaneous T-cell lymphoma.

β-Caryophyllene and β-caryophyllene oxide are potent anti-inflammatory agents against lymphoma cells. *Appendix B: Taming Cytokines* has some additional ideas on lowering inflammatory cytokines.

8.11 Cancers of the Brain and Nervous System

Killing Cells

Most brain tumors are metastases from lung cancer, breast cancer, melanoma, etc. Cancers that arise within the central nervous system are referred to as primary CNS tumors. Most primary tumors are gliomas — cancers of the glial cells. These cells nourish the neurons. The deadliest gliomas are glioblastomas.

CBD kills glioma cancer cells via apoptosis in both in vitro and animal xenograft studies.

THC kills glioblastoma cells, and THC + CBD works better than either THC or CBD alone.

β-Caryophyllene inhibits the proliferation of glioblastoma cells.

Controlling Inflammatory Cytokines

TGF-β exerts strong immunosuppressive effects in gliomas, but there is a lack of information on how cannabis compounds might help. See *Appendix B: Taming Cytokines*.

Controlling Gene Expression

CBD lowers the ID1 oncogene, thereby reducing the invasiveness of glioblastomas.

8.12 Stomach Cancer

Killing Cancer Cells

β-caryophyllene oxide is cytotoxic against cell lines for stomach cancer. Additionally, β-caryophyllene oxide has increased the cytotoxicity for cancer cells of doxorubicin while decreasing its toxicity for normal cells.

d-Limonene, menthol, and linalool kill stomach cancer cells. Apigenin is also cytotoxic.

Controlling Cytokines

IL-6 is elevated in stomach cancer. Its levels continue to rise as cancer progresses, promoting angiogenesis. IL-22 is elevated in stomach cancer. TGF-β is elevated in stomach cancer, and high levels indicate a poor prognosis for patients with advanced cancer.

The Helicobacter Pylori bacteria increases the risk of gastric cancer by stimulating the production of TNF-α and IL-1β.

For general ideas on controlling cytokines, see *Appendix B: Taming Cytokines*.

8.13 Melanoma and Other Skin Cancers

Killing Cancer Cells

CBD and THC induce apoptosis by different mechanisms in melanoma cells. THC + CBD in a 1/1 ratio is even more effective against melanoma in both in vitro experiments and animal studies. CBG exhibits significant inhibitory activity against mouse skin melanoma cells.

Linalool and β-caryophyllene are cytotoxic against human melanoma cells. 4-Terpineol is cytotoxic against murine melanoma cells, including drug-resistant cells. γ-Terpinene is cytotoxic against mouse melanoma cells,

α-Pinene, used as the main component of a fragrant environment, has reduced melanoma tumor size in mice by about 40%. However, the same effect was not observed in an in vitro experiment, suggesting that the effect of the fragrant environment was indirect.

α-humulene kills human melanoma cells.

Halting Cell Division

4-Terpineol induces cell-cycle arrest in murine mesothelioma and B16 melanoma.

Controlling Cytokines

IL-1β, IFN-γ, and CXCL10 are significantly increased in advanced melanoma patients. IL-8 is essential for cancer growth.

In a mouse model, IL1-β was required for tumor invasiveness and angiogenesis. Interestingly, a blockade of IL-1 inhibited melanoma metastasis to some locations but not others. Metastases to bone marrow, spleen, liver, lung, pancreas, skeletal muscle, adrenal gland, and heart were inhibited by IL-1 blockade. Yet, metastases to the kidney, testis, brain, skin, and gastrointestinal tract were not inhibited.

In a mouse model of melanoma, IL-23 stimulated the production of IL-17, which stimulated the production of IL-6, which stimulated tumor growth. Lowering any of these cytokines led to a reduction in tumor growth.

For general ideas on controlling cytokines, see *Appendix B: Taming Cytokines.*

8.14 Ovarian Cancer

Killing Cancer Cells

α-Pinene is cytotoxic against human epithelial ovarian cancer. Cystadenocarcinoma is a malignant cyst derived from glandular epithelium. 1,8-Cineole, α-pinene, and β-pinene may induce apoptosis in Cystadenocarcinomas.

Cisplatin is used to treat metastatic ovarian cancer after other treatment strategies have failed. CBD helps repair cisplatin-induced liver damage in mice.

Controlling Inflammatory Cytokines

IL-1β promotes ovarian cancer. Elevated IL-1β in ovarian cancer epithelial cells is inversely correlated with overall survival. IL-6 has promoted tumor growth and angiogenesis in ovarian cancer in a clinical study. Suppression of IL-6 had a beneficial effect.

TNF-α stimulated the production of IL-17 and promoted tumor growth in a mouse model of ovarian cancer. Suppression of TNF-α via the drug infliximab substantially reduced IL-17 levels and responsiveness to IL-1 and IL-23.

Malignant ovarian tumors produce significant amounts of TNF-α, which generates IL-6 and promotes tumor growth and proliferation. Without TNF-α, the same tumors become noninvasive and show high levels of apoptosis. These results are based on several human ovarian tumors grown in female mice.

See *Appendix B: Taming Cytokines* regarding the suppression of IL-1β, IL-6, TNF-α, IL-17, and IL-23.

8.15 Cancers of the Oral Cavity, Pharynx, and Esophagus

Killing Cancer Cells

CBG kills Human Oral Epithelial cancer Cells, including multi-drug resistant cells. Linalool is cytotoxic against oral cancer cells.

Perillyl alcohol and perillic acid are metabolites of d-limonene. These two compounds improve the effectiveness of radiation against tongue squamous cell cancer and pharynx squamous cell cancer. The pharynx is a complex collection of structures extending above and below the back of the mouth.

Inhibiting Invasion and Metastasis

Menthol has reduced the invasion potential of oral squamous carcinoma cell lines.

Cytokine Control

TNF-α promotes the development of pre-cancerous cells leading to oral squamous cell cancer. IL-1β promotes malignant transformation and tumor aggressiveness in oral cancer.

Geraniol lowers TNF-α and IL-1β in a rat model of tongue cancer. *Appendix B: Taming Cytokines* has some additional ideas on taming these two cytokines.

8.16 Other Cancers

Thyroid Cancer. Apigenin promotes apoptosis in thyroid cancer cells.

Bone Cancer. Linalool is cytotoxic against bone cancer cells (Osteosarcoma Epithelial Cells).

Fibrosarcoma is a highly metastatic form of bone cancer that expresses the cytokine TNF-α. A form of this cancer is found in mice. When mice with the cancer were treated with mouse-derived TNF-α, metastatic tumors sprang up more quickly. But when TNF-α was neutralized, the rate of new metastatic tumor creation slowed down. See *Appendix B: Taming Cytokines*.

Neuroblastoma is a childhood cancer originating in the sympathetic nervous system. CBD reduces the invasiveness of treated tumor cells and triggers apoptosis. Terpinolene prevents cell proliferation in mouse neuroblastoma. BCP and BCPO also induce apoptosis in neuroblastoma cells.

Cancers in the region of the kidneys. Linalool is cytotoxic against renal cancers.

Metastatic Testicular Cancer. CBD helps repair cisplatin-induced liver damage in mice. Cisplatin is used to treat metastatic testicular and bladder cancer after other treatment strategies have failed.

Thymus cancer. THC induces apoptosis.

Spleen cancer. THC induces apoptosis.

9: Visualizing the Research

In the following Summary table, medical specialties run across the top row. Cannabis compounds run down the left column. The compounds include nine cannabinoids, nineteen terpenes, and one flavonoid. The cannabinoids are labeled with acronyms.

Some of the table cells contain acronyms whose meanings are as follows:

INV – in vitro study

AN - animal study

SS - small-scale human study

When an acronym occurs in a cell, it acknowledges research in that area. For example, the cell for CBD and arthritis acknowledges CBD's use in treating arthritis

Several things pop out from these tables. There are no large-scale studies. Of the conditions investigated, chemical addiction appears to be the least studied. Pain has the most cannabinoids. By contrast, the use of terpenes in treating arthritis has been strongly emphasized. Almost all of the cancer research has been in vitro.

Finally, consider the significance for strain developers. Or example, to get a strain that's good for cardiovascular conditions, an excellent initial goal would be to develop a strain with adequate amounts of CBD, THC, BCP, and perhaps THCV, as well as terpenes such as d-limonene, linalool, and eucalyptol.

Compounds and Conditions

	Arthritis	Pain & Nausea	Neurological Conditions	Psychiatric Conditions	Chemical Addictions	Cardiovascular Conditions	Cancer
CBD	AN	SS	SS	SS	SS	SS	INV
CBDA		AN					INV
THC	SS	SS	SS	SS	SS	SS	AN
THCA		AN	INV				
CBC		AN	AN	AN			
CBG		AN	AN				
CBN		AN	IV	AN			
THCV		AN	AN			INV	
Δ^8-THC		SS					
BCP	AN	AN	AN	AN	SS	AN	INV
BCPO	INV	AN			SS		INV
Geraniol	AN						INV
d-Limonene	AN			AN		AN	INV
Terpinolene				AN		INV	INV

Compounds and Conditions (continued)

	Arthritis	Pain & Nausea	Neurological Conditions	Psychiatric Conditions	Chemical Addictions	Cardiovascular Conditions	Cancer
α-Pinene	INV		INV	AN			INV
α-Humulene	AN	AN					INV
Linalool	INV	AN	AN	SS		AN	INV
Guaiol	INV						
α-Bisabolol		AN					INV
Nerolidol	AN						INV
Terpineol	INV						INV
Eucalyptol	AN	AN	INV	SS		AN	
α-Terpinene	INV						
γ-Terpinene						INV	
Borneol							INV
β-Eudesmol	INV						INV
Menthol							INV
Valencene							INV
Apigenin	INV		AN	AN			INV

A: Common Cannabis Compounds

The compounds in the following list were chosen based on their prevalence in the Connecticut Medical Marijuana Registry. Information on which strains contain these various compounds is taken from the Registry and an associated strain-name guide. Additional information on specific compounds is, unless otherwise specified, taken from Wikipedia.

As of this writing, there have been no large-scale studies on the use of individual cannabis compounds. Information on cross-reactions with other medications is lacking—caveat emptor.

Cannabinoids

Naturally occurring cannabinoids are found only in the cannabis species, the one possible exception being β-Caryophyllene. Cannabis plants are classified as marijuana or hemp according to whether they contain significant amounts of THC.

Cannabidiol – CBD. Plentiful in heat-treated flowers of hemp and marijuana strains bred for high CBD content. CBD is largely free of adverse effects but has been known to cause diarrhea.

Cannabidiolic Acid – CBDA. Plentiful in the raw flowers of hemp and marijuana strains bred for high CBD content.

Δ^9-Tetrahydrocannabinol – THC, Δ^9-THC. Plentiful in heat-treated flowers of most marijuana strains.

Δ^9-Teahydrocannabinolic Acid – THCA. Plentiful in raw flowers of most marijuana strains.

Cannabichromene – CBC. Moderate amounts in lemon skunk, Theraplant's 360X.

Cannabigerol – CBG. Moderate amounts in Sour Diesel, Theraplant's 360X, Lemon Skunk.

Cannabigerolic Acid – CBGA. Small amounts in Wedding Cake, Lemon Skunk.

Cannabinol – CBN. Small amounts in Theraplant's 360X, Lemon Skunk.

Δ^9*-teahydrocannabivarin – THCV.* Small amounts in Lemon Skunk

Δ^8*-Teahydrocannabinol – Δ^8-THC.* Trace amounts are found in most cannabis strains. It is mostly derived chemically from CBD and similar compounds. Δ^8-THC is intoxicating but less so than Δ^9-THC. It is legal at the Federal level.

Terpenes

Generally speaking, pure 100% terpenes may irritate the skin of those who are sensitive, and they tend to be lethal if they enter the airways. Reputable commercial products specify their potency, and reputable 100% products come with a warning and a suggested dilution, usually 1% for internal use.

Most terpenes have human uses — in cosmetics, as a flavoring in foods and beverages, and as scents in household cleaning products.

β-Caryophyllene – BCP. Isomers include *trans-caryophyllene* and *(E)-Caryophyllene.* BCP is plentiful in most cannabis strains. It is also found in cloves, hops, basil, oregano, black pepper, and the balm of Gilead. BCP is widely used as a flavoring agent. In moderation, it smells a bit like black pepper. It absorbs slowly when used topically (personal observation).

β-Caryophyllene Oxide – BCPO. Trace amounts occur in most marijuana strains. Also found in cloves, hops, basil, oregano, black pepper, and the balm of Gilead.

β-Myrcene. Plentiful in Blue Dream, Sour Diesel, Ace of Spades. Moderate amounts are found in Dutch Treat, Connecticut Pharmaceutical's Rubidex, Tickle Kush. It is also found in wild thyme, hops, mangoes, and cardamom. The FDA has banned myrcene's use as a food additive on the grounds that it is carcinogenic[myrcene-fda]. As a result, β-myrcene has been dropped from this work's analyses.

β-Pinene. Plentiful in ACDC, Cold Creek Kush, Green Kush; moderate amounts in White Shark. It is also found in cumin, hops, cluster pine, and horsewood.

Geraniol (not be confused with geranial). Plentiful in Dutch Treat. Also found in citrus fruits, rose oil, palmarosa oil, and citronella oil.

d-Limonene, also known as *(+)-Limonene* , *(R)-(+)-Limonene,* and *(+)-carvene.* Benefits are largely attributable to metabolites such as *perillyl alcohol* and *perillic acid.* Moderate amounts in Sour Diesel, Wedding Cake. It is found mainly in citrus fruits. d-Limonene is the active ingredient in citrus degreasers; it can be a mild skin irritant. It is readily absorbed when used topically (personal observation).

Terpinolene, also known as *δ-terpinene.* Moderate amounts in Ace of Spades, Ghost Train. Also found in cumin and in the leaves of the melaleuca tree (tea tree).

α-Pinene. Moderate amounts in Green Kush. Also found in conifers, ironwort, and sage. Smells like pine if not too concentrated. It is readily absorbed when used topically (personal observation).

Phytol. Moderate amounts in Blue Dream, Sour Diesel. Also found in jasmine flowers, green tea, and wild lettuce. Small amounts are in virtually all plants as a decomposition product of chlorophyll.

α-Humulene , also known as α-caryophyllene. Small amounts in Wedding Cake, Thunderstruck, Green Kush, Pedro's Sweet Sativa, Connecticut Pharmaceuticals' Somnidex, and Lemon Skunk. Also found in hops, sage, ginseng, spearmint, and ginger.

Linalool. Small amounts in Wedding Cake. Also found in orange, lavender, and coriander.

Guaiol, also known as *champacol.* Small amounts in Wedding Cake. Also found in oil of guaiacum, cypress pine.

Ocimene. Small amounts in Connecticut Pharmaceuticals' Somnidex. Also found in mint, parsley, basil, mangoes, and orchids.

α-Bisabolol. Small amounts in Green Kush. Also found in German chamomile and the bark of the Brazilian candeia tree.

Nerolidol comes in two isomorphic forms, *trans-nerolidol* and *cis-Nerolidol*. Small amounts in San Fernando Valley. Also found in blossoms of the bitter orange tree and in ginger, jasmine, and lavender.

Terpineol. Isomers include *α-terpineol* , *β-terpineol* , *γ-terpineol* , and *4-terpineol* (aka *terpinen-4-ol*). Trace amounts in Wedding Cake. Also found in lilacs, lime oil, pine trees, eucalyptus, and the leaves of melaleuca trees.

Eucalyptol, also known as *1,8-cineole*. Trace amounts in most marijuana strains. Also found in camphor, great basin sagebrush, and eucalyptus. It is readily absorbed when used topically (personal observation).

α-Terpinene. Trace amounts in most strains of marijuana. Also found in coriander, lemon, and cumin.

γ-Terpinene. Trace amounts in most marijuana strains. Also found in citrus fruits, coriander, cumin, and European centaury.

Borneol. Trace amounts in most marijuana strains. Also found in the essential oils of valerian, chamomile, and lavender.

β-Eudesmol. Trace amounts in most strains of marijuana. Also found in Cng zhú rhizomes, the warionia shrub, and the Japanese mountain yam.

Isopulegol. Trace amounts in most strains of marijuana. Also found in lemon balm, orange peel, corn mint, and peppermint.

p-Cymene. Trace amounts in some strains of marijuana. Also found in anise, coriander, cumin, thyme, mace, oregano, and eucalyptus.

Camphene. Trace amounts in most cannabis strains. Also found in dill, caraway, hyssop, and fennel.

Sabinene. Trace amounts in most marijuana strains. Also found in Norway spruce, black pepper, and nutmeg.

Menthol. Trace amounts in most strains. Also found in peppermint, corn mint, and spearmint.

α-Phellandrene. Trace amounts in most strains. Also found in turmeric leaf, allspice, and eucalyptus oil.

Valencene. Trace amounts in most strains. Also found in Valencia oranges.

Apigenin is a flavonoid rather than a terpene. Trace amounts occur in most cannabis strains. Apigenin is also found in parsley, celery, celeriac, and chamomile tea.

The following compounds were not used in the analysis of compounds and conditions but have been included here for completeness: CBGA, β-pinene, β-myrcene, ocimene, isopulegol, p-cymene, camphene, sabinene, and α-phellandrene.

Additional Resources

Medical Marijuana Brand Registry. Department of Consumer Protection. The State of Connecticut. Online 2015 Mar 24 and later.

Connecticut Medical Marijuana Strain Name Guide. Rahn B. Leafy. Updated 2019 March 5.

Ct Medical Marijuana Strain Listing. Unattributed. Ct Medical Marijuana Critic. Undated.

FDA Removes 7 Synthetic Flavoring Substances from Food Additives List. Center for Food Safety and Applied Nutrition. FDA. 2018 October 5.

B: Taming Cytokines

Inflammatory cytokines may be of short-term benefit in fighting injury and infection. But inflammation comes at a cost and can have negative consequences.

Cannabis compounds are well-known for controlling inflammatory cytokines, which is what accounts for much of their value in treating conditions such as arthritis, inflammatory pain, and many cancers.

This appendix enumerates key cytokines and what's known about the cannabis compounds that are able to inhibit them.

Lowering IL-6

CBD, THC, perillyl alcohol, α-terpineol, 4-terpineol, eucalyptol, and apigenin may help lower IL-6.

CBD lowers IL-6 in ischemic rat hearts and in chemically stressed mouse microglial cells. THC reduces IL-6 in chemically stressed macrophages and in mouse microglial cell lines. BCP lowers IL-6, IL-1β, and TNF-α in a microglial cell line used to study neuroinflammation.

Perillyl alcohol, a metabolite of d-limonene, lowers IL-6, IL-1β, and TNF-α in a rat model of stroke. α-Terpineol lowers IL-6 in human cheek cells stressed with desiccated orange juice. α-Terpineol and 4-terpineol (aka terpinen-4-ol) lower both IL-6 and IL-1β in chemically stressed human macrophages. Eucalyptol has lowered IL-6, IL-1β, and TNF-α in various in vitro and animal models of inflammation. The flavonoid apigenin lowers IL-6 in chemically stressed mice.

Lowering IL-1

CBD, THC, BCP (β-caryophyllene), nerolidol, perillyl alcohol (and thus d-limonene), eucalyptol, α-Humulene, and geraniol may all help lower IL-1.

CBD and THC lower IL-1β in chemically stressed mouse microglial cells. CBD lowers IL1-β and TNF-α in a mouse model of multiple sclerosis. BCP (β-caryophyllene) lowers IL-1β and TNF-α in in vitro tests.

Nerolidol inhibits IL1-β and TNF-α in mouse peritonitis. As noted above, perillyl alcohol reduced IL-1β and TNF-α in a rat model of stroke, and eucalyptol lowered IL-1.

α-Humulene lowered IL-1β and TNF-α in rat paw edema. Geraniol lowered IL-1β and TNF-α in rat tongue cancer.

Lowering TNF-α

CBD, BCP (β-caryophyllene), nerolidol, perillyl alcohol, α-humulene, eucalyptol, α-terpineol, geraniol, and apigenin may all help lower TNF-α.

As noted above, CBD, BCP, nerolidol, perillyl alcohol, α-humulene, eucalyptol, α-terpineol, and geraniol all lower TNF-α.

The flavonoid apigenin lowered TNF-α in an experiential model of mouse pancreatitis. Apigenin lowered TNF-α and upregulated the anti-inflammatory cytokine IL-10 in mouse leukemia macrophages.

Lowering IL-17

CBD, THC, and BCP (β-caryophyllene) may help lower IL-17.

CBD lowers IL-17, as does THC. JWH-133 lowers IL-17 in macrophages, so the same is likely true of the stronger CB2 agonist BCP.

Lowering IL-8

THCA inhibits IL-8 in inflamed colon tissues.

Lowering GM-CSF and CCL3

CBD lowers GM-CSF and CCL3 in triple-negative breast cancer.

Lowering Nitric Oxide

α-Humulene, α-terpinene, α-pinene, and β-pinene neutralize the free radical nitric oxide. d-Limonene also lowers nitric oxide levels.

Nitric oxide is, of course, not a cytokine, but it may be worth tamping down due to its role in inflammatory processes. Caution may be merited, however. It functions as a neurotransmitter at neuron synapses. It induces vasodilatation in the cardiovascular system. And it plays a role in immune response where cytokine-activated macrophages release nitric oxide in high concentrations.

C: Cannabis History and Terminology

The evolution of cannabis goes back 28 million years to the eastern Tibetan Plateau. The original strains appear to have been more hemp than marijuana. Chinese farmers used cannabis for oil, rope, clothing, and paper four thousand years ago. Two thousand seven hundred years ago, shamans were using cannabis to get high.

The Historic Rise and Fall of Cannabis

Knowledge of medical cannabis came to Europe in the 19th century, mainly through the efforts of Sir. William Brooke O'Shaughnessy. He observed its use in India, did experiments, published his research, brought quantities of cannabis specimens and seeds to Briton, and inspired pharmacies to carry cannabis tinctures.

Cannabis, including industrial hemp, was effectively driven underground in the United States in 1937 by the Marihuana Tax Act. The act was primarily the brainchild of Harry Anslinger, the founding commissioner of the Federal Bureau of Narcotics. He sold the idea with purported cases of stoned black men raping young white women and the like.

Time Out for Some Terminology

Cannabis is both a species and a genus. The species contains three well-known wild *varieties*: Cannabis Sativa, Cannabis Indica, and Cannabis Ruderalis. They all readily interbreed. Standard botanical conventions force them into the same species. A great many cultivars have resulted from interbreeding the wild varieties.

In 1937, nobody knew about CBD and THC. But there was a distinction in usage. Hemp was cannabis used for rope, cloth, and oil. Marijuana was cannabis used to get high.

Roger Adams in the U.S and Lord Todd in the U.K. first extracted CBD from cannabis in 1940. Loewe, Wollner, Matchett, and Levine extracted THC from cannabis in 1942.

The official boundary between hemp and marijuana was set in 2018 by the 2018 farm bill. Cannabis strains with less than 0.3% THC are hemp, and the others are marijuana. This distinction is now universal among growers, merchants, and users.

Today, "marijuana" is still a dirty word to many. There is a trend to use "cannabis" as a polite synonym for marijuana even though hemp plants are cannabis plants.

Modern Research and Repression

Dr. Raphael Mechoulam first isolated THC from cannabis and determined its structure in 1964. Israel awarded him the state's highest cultural honor for his cannabis research in 2001 — the Israel Prize. The twenty years following Dr. Mechoulam's achievement led to many discoveries, including the ability of cannabis to stimulate appetite, dampen nausea, quell seizures, relieve pain, and even stop an asthma attack in seconds rather than minutes.

In the meantime, Congress replaced the Tax Act with the Controlled Substances Act of 1970. This act banned cannabis altogether, and the era of mass incarceration began. In 1988, a new three-strikes law mandated life imprisonment for chronic cannabis users. At that time, all government-funded cannabis research was devoted to substantiating the adverse effects of marijuana.

Some of this government research led to a significant breakthrough in 1988. Working in Dr. Allyn Howlett's laboratory at the St. Louis University Medical School, a graduate student, William Anthony Devane, discovered cannabinoid receptors—cell membrane receptors activated by THC. The discovery of cannabinoid receptors inspired new research the world over. Investigators learned that most cannabinoid receptors were of two types, CB1 and CB2.

CB1 is found mainly in the central nervous system and the lungs, liver, kidneys, and white blood cells. CB2 is located in the immune system, the red bone marrow that produces blood cells, and the peripheral nerve terminals, where its activation relieves pain. CB2 is also found throughout the gut.

The discovery of cannabinoid receptors led to the idea of cannabinoids. They are chemicals that are either structurally similar to THC or that bind to cannabinoid receptors. CBD qualifies as a cannabinoid through its structural similarity to THC. The terpene β-caryophyllene qualifies as a cannabinoid because it binds strongly to CB2 receptors.

Researchers wondered why brains and bodies should have receptors for THC and other cannabinoids. They guessed there had to be as yet undiscovered internally created cannabinoids whose purpose was to bind to the cannabinoid receptors. In other words, there had to exist *endocannabinoids*. The first such was discovered in 1992 by chemists Ondřej Hanuš and William Anthony Devane. They named it anandamide after the Sanskrit word for bliss.

Anandamide binds to the same CB1 and CB2 receptors as THC. CBD and THC raise anandamide levels. Another endocannabinoid goes by the acronym 2-AG. It also binds to both CB1 and CB2.

Can anandamide get people high? No, it is metabolized so quickly that nobody will get high on it. However, some people have less of the

FAAH enzyme that degrades anandamide. Such people have a gene variant that causes lower levels of FAAH to be produced, resulting in higher levels of anandamide. We know anandamide is an upper because this gene variant is more prevalent in countries with happier people. This key to happiness counts even more than having a great climate, which is also valuable.

World Cannabis Legality

Today, in 2022, recreational cannabis is still illegal in most of the world.

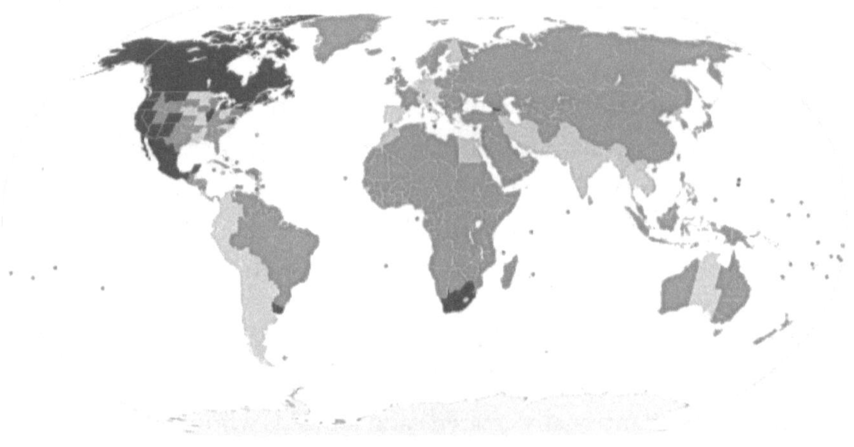

D: Environmental Neurotoxins

The following list presents neurotoxins in approximate order of decreasing risk, where risk is the likelihood of being poisoned times the resulting damage in case of being poisoned. However, risk varies depending on geographical location, economic status, and ethnicity. Also, males tend to be more sensitive to neurotoxins than females.

- *Poisonous metals*
  - Aluminum damages the blood-brain barrier, impairs learning, and reduces motor coordination; it has a causal role in autism spectrum disorder, brain aging, and Alzheimer's disease. Exposure is mainly the result of sociopolitical factors.
  - Mercury contributes to autistic behaviors. It can result in impaired neurological development in infants and children. It can cause central nervous system damage, depression, behavioral disturbances, deafness, and visual field constriction. The most common source of mercury poisoning is seafood. The losses due to mercury and aluminum are additive.
  - Manganese. Chronic exposure has been shown to produce a parkinsonism-like illness. Children may develop increased hyperactive and oppositional behavior. Well-water is a primary source of exposure. Another source is the synthetic analog of khat, methcathinone. Street names include "Jeff," "Mulka," "Murtsovka," "Cat," "M-Cat," and "Ephedrone."
  - Cadmium plays a causal role in autism spectrum disorder.
  - So does Lead.

- Arsenic occurs in everyday foods such as apple juice, grape juice, and rice.
- Depleted uranium is a known neurotoxin; its primary environmental source is the U.S. military.
- Zinc-induced copper deficiency. Zinc itself isn't toxic, but it does flush copper, and the resulting deficiency can result in loss of the myelin sheath surrounding nerve axons, causing widespread neuropathies. Vitamin B12 deficiency causes similar problems.

- Poisonous chemicals
  - Ethel alcohol. Long-term use causes brain damage.
  - Methanol and formaldehyde. The liver metabolizes methyl alcohol to formaldehyde, which is a carcinogenic toxin. The human body has a limited ability to process formaldehyde. Airborne formaldehyde causes allergies and asthma.
  - Fluoride is a neurotoxin that is especially harmful to children.
  - Chlorpyrifos is a neurotoxin that is used as a commercial pesticide. There is no known safe exposure level. Children are especially vulnerable. The question of whether to ban it has been in the courts and EPA reviews for many years.
  - Tetrachloroethylene is a solvent used in dry cleaning. Chronic exposure may cause impaired cognitive and motor performance.
  - Aspirin causes hearing loss. It also decreases word discrimination and temporal integration ability.
  - MSG may contribute to fibromyalgia.

- Biological toxins. Sources include C. botulinum, C. tetani, pufferfish, poisonous snakes, curare, and the deathstalker scorpion.

E: Glossary of Medical Terms

Acetylcholine. A neurotransmitter that plays an essential role in forming and preserving memories.

Acetylcholinesterase. The enzyme responsible for breaking down the neurotransmitter acetylcholine.

Allele. A SNP variant.

Alzheimer's disease. A progressive form of presenile dementia characterized by impaired memory followed by impaired thought and speech, and finally, complete helplessness.

Amygdala. A region located deep within the temporal lobes of the brain's cerebrum. The amygdala plays a primary role in processing memory, decision-making, and emotional responses.

Anandamide. The first endocannabinoid to be discovered.

Angiogenesis. The process by which tissues stimulate the growth of new blood vessels.

Anorexia. An eating disorder governed by an overpowering desire to be thin.

Anterior cingulate gyrus. A brain region involved in attention allocation, reward anticipation, decision-making, ethics and morality, impulse control, and emotion.

Anxiety. Inner turmoil and unpleasant feelings of dread over anticipated events.

Apoptosis (also known as *programmed cell death*). *Cellular* self-destruction.

Arthritis. A chronic inflammation of joints.

Atherosclerosis. A buildup of abnormal fatty deposits and fibrous tissue in the inner layer of the arteries.

Autism spectrum disorder. A neurological and developmental disorder that affects how people interact with others, communicate, learn, and behave. Symptoms begin to appear within the first two years of life.

Autonomic nervous system. A control system that regulates bodily functions such as the heart rate, digestion, respiratory rate, pupillary response, urination, and sexual arousal. This system is the primary mechanism in control of the fight-or-flight response.

Benzodiazepines. A class of drugs used to treat panic, anxiety, insomnia, seizures, and alcohol withdrawal.

Bipolar disorder. A mood disorder characterized by periods of depression and periods of abnormally-elevated energy or happiness.

Cachexia. A syndrome resulting in muscle protein loss.

Cannabinoid receptor. A cell-membrane receptor that interacts with THC, specifically, either of the receptors, CB1 or CB2.

Cannabinoid. A compound that interacts with the cannabinoid receptors or is structurally similar to compounds that do.

Cannabis compound. A cannabinoid, terpene, or flavonoid found in cannabis plants.

Cannabis indica, Cannabis sativa, Cannabis ruderalis. Native cannabis strains found in the wild.

Cannabis. A plant belonging to the species C. sativa. Also, any plant product harvested from cannabis plants. The term cannabis is often used as a euphemism for marijuana, but hemp plants also belong to this same species.

Case study. A scientific study of a patient's personal story.

CB1, CB2. See Cannabinoid receptor.

Cell-cycle arrest. Preventing a cell from reproducing. This can happen at any stage of a cell's life cycle.

Chemical addiction. Involvement with a chemical such that attempted cessation leads to the discovery that stopping is easier said than done. Further evidence of addiction is that use has caused problems severe enough to impair health, work, and personal relationships.

CNR1 gene. The gene that codes for the CB1 cannabinoid receptor.

Cytotoxic. Toxic to cells.

Depression. A mental and behavioral disorder characterized by a loss of interest or a loss of feeling of pleasure in activities that usually bring joy to people.

Dyslipidemia. Abnormal levels of lipids — such as cholesterol and triglycerides — in the blood. It can involve HDL levels that are too low or LDL levels that are too high.

Endocannabinoid. Endogenous neurotransmitters that originate within the body and bind to cannabinoid receptors.

Epilepsy. A group of non-communicable neurological disorders characterized by recurrent epileptic seizures — periods of unusual behavior, sensations, and sometimes loss of awareness.

Essential tremor. A condition that involves shaking of hands and other extremities.

FAAH gene. The gene responsible for breaking down the endocannabinoid anandamide.

Fibromyalgia. A medical condition defined by the presence of widespread chronic pain, fatigue, waking unrefreshed, cognitive symptoms, lower abdominal pain or cramps, and depression.

Flavonoids. Water-soluble pigmented antioxidants found in most plants.

Fragile X syndrome. The result of an inherited genetic defect in a gene that protects against mental retardation.

Genotype. A pair of alleles.

Glaucoma. A group of eye diseases that damage the optic nerve and cause vision loss.

Heart attack (myocardial infarction). A sudden blockage of blood flow to a part of the heart muscle.

Hemorrhagic Stroke. A stroke caused by a ruptured blood vessel in the brain.

Hemp. Cannabis with less than 0.3% THC.

Huntington's disease. An inherited genetic illness that causes premature death of brain neurons in the striatum, which coordinates movement, and in the frontal cortex, which controls thinking and emotions.

Il-1. Interleukin-1, a family of pro-inflammatory cytokines.

IL-17. Interleukin-17, a family of pro-inflammatory cytokines.

IL-6. Interleukin-6, a pro-inflammatory cytokine.

IL-8. Interleukin-8, a pro-inflammatory cytokine.

In vitro study. The results of laboratory experiments with cells or tissues taken from plants, animals, or humans.

Inflammation. A local response to cellular injury that initiates the elimination of noxious agents or damaged tissue.

Intoxicating. Exciting or stupefying with possible loss of physical and mental control.

Invasion. A tumor spreading to a nearby location.

Ischemic stroke. A stroke caused by the narrowing or blockage of a blood vessel supplying the brain.

Large-scale study. A study of more than a thousand patients. Such a study involves careful attention to experimental design to avoid experimental errors.

Marijuana. Cannabis with at least 0.3% THC.

Metastasis. A tumor spreading to a distant location.

Migraine. A disorder characterized by recurrent moderate to severe headaches.

Multiple sclerosis. A neurological condition in which the insulating covers of nerve cells in the brain and spinal cord are damaged.

Mutation. Any event that changes genetic structure.

Myocardial ischemia. Reduced blood flow to the heart.

Myocarditis. Inflammation of the heart muscle.

Nausea. A diffuse sense of unease often perceived as an urge to vomit.

Necrosis. Cell death caused by events outside of the cell.

Neurogenesis. The process of adding new nerve cells to the nervous system.

Neuropathic pain. Pain that originates within the nervous system itself.

Neurotransmitter. A signaling molecule secreted by a neuron to affect another neuron across a synapse.

Nociceptive pain. Pain that responds to damaging or potentially damaging physical stimulation. Such pain is initiated by pain receptors known as nociceptors.

Osteoarthritis. A degenerative joint disease that results from the breakdown of joint cartilage and underlying bone.

Panic. Sudden, overpowering fright and extreme anxiety.

Parkinson's disease. A disease caused by the die-off of dopamine-producing neurons that supply parts of the brain involved in movement and reward.

Post-Traumatic Stress Disorder (PTSD). Residual feelings of stress or fright experienced even when one is no longer in danger.

Prions—misfolded proteins capable of replication.

Psychoactive. Affecting mood, perception, cognition, mind, or behavior.

Psychomimetic. Producing effects that resemble psychotic symptoms.

Psychotropic. Acting on the mind.

Rheumatoid arthritis. A long-term autoimmune disorder in which the immune system attacks the synovial membranes that hold the fluid that lubricates the joints.

Schizophrenia. A mental illness involving three kids of problems:

- positive symptoms - experiencing what is not there (hallucinations)
- negative symptoms - not experiencing what is there
- cognitive symptoms - thinking problems

Single nucleotide polymorphism (SNP). A location within a gene with genetic variation. SNPs normally come in pairs, with one inherited from the mother and one from the father.

Small-scale study, small-scale trial. A study of fewer than a thousand subjects. Small-scale studies divide patients into different treatment groups based on varying criteria.

Stress. Psychological pain involving feelings of strain and pressure.

Stroke. A sudden interruption of blood flow to the brain.

Terpenes. Light-weight oily compounds found not only in cannabis but in most other plants.

Tincture. A compound dissolved in alcohol or oil.

TNF-α. Tumor necrosis factor-alpha, a pro-inflammatory cytokine involved in inflammatory responses to infection.

Tourette Syndrome. A nervous system condition causes people to have involuntary tics—sudden twitches, movements, or sounds that people repeatedly do.

Typical pain. See nociceptive pain.

Xenograft. A technique in which tissue of one species is grafted onto an organism of a different species. An example would be grafting lung tumors into a mouse with no immune system.

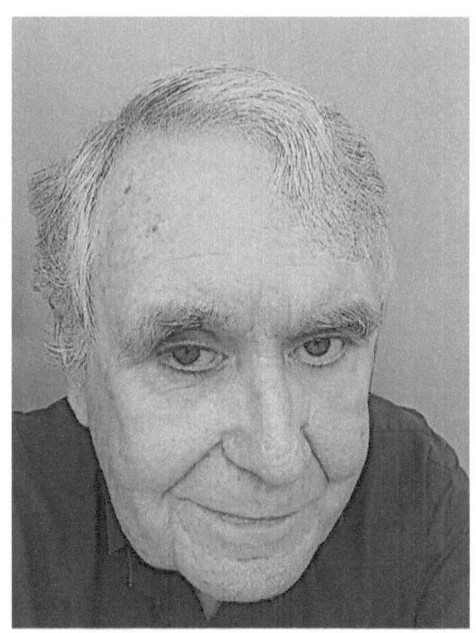

About the Author

Jim Williams grew up in Southern California, in Poway and Escondido, just north of San Diego.

At Carleton College, Jim studied math and physics and was taught how scientists think. And he longed for the Southern California sunshine. At U.C. Berkeley, Jim lived two blocks from the Oakland Black Panther headquarters and learned about blacks' problems with cops. And he got a Ph.D. in mathematics.

At Berkeley and later at BGSU and the MITRE Corporation, Jim published research in topology, algebra, category theory, logic, automated deduction, information security, and the integrity of medical information systems.

After retiring, Jim became curious why his doctors thought medical marijuana could help with his prostate cancer. He learned that CBD, THC, and a dozen other cannabis compounds are relevant to serious illness.

The result is a book on cannabis compounds for medical conditions such as arthritis, intractable pain, Alzheimer's disease, schizophrenia, alcoholism, heart disease, and cancer.

In writing citations and references for the book, Jim developed a groundbreaking citation architecture that features citations whose references show up as mouseover notes. The notes are annotated with icons automatically gleaned from links to the referenced works.

Read more at https://hempforhealth.net/.